AlvinAiley®
dance moves!

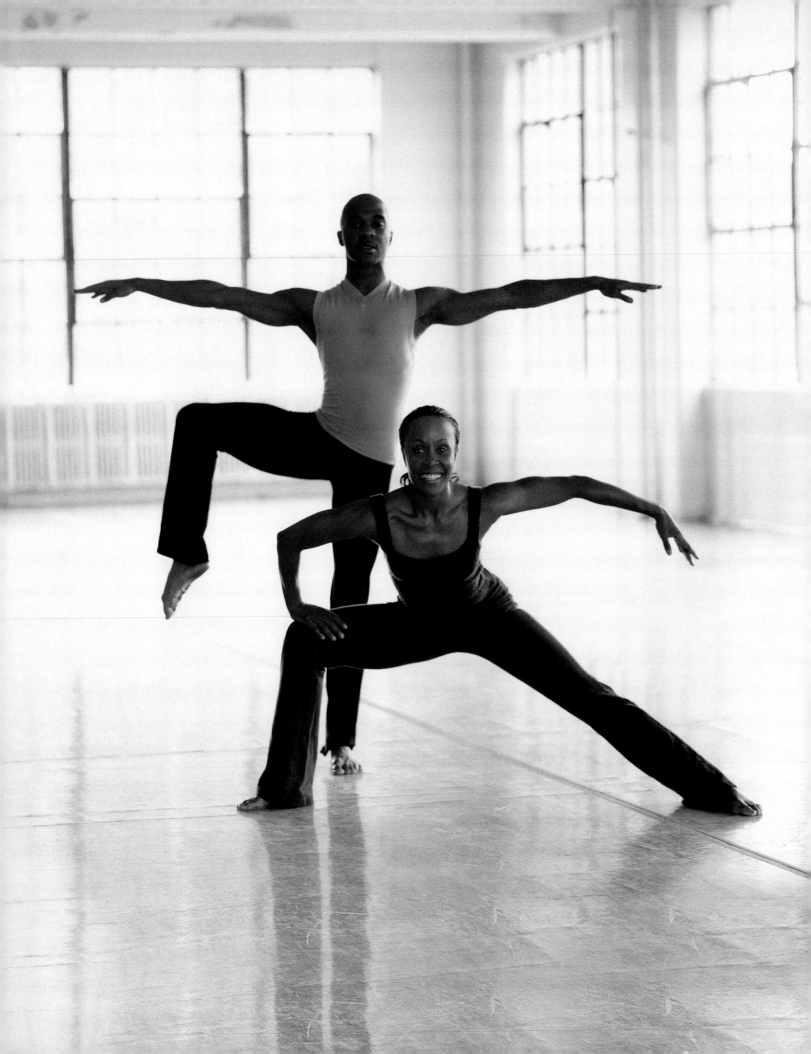

AlvinAiley®
dance moves!

a new
way to
exercise

LISE FRIEDMAN

photographs by CHRIS CALLIS

Stewart, Tabori & Chang ◆ New York

Published in 2003 by Stewart, Tabori, & Chang
A Company of La Martinière Groupe
115 West 18th Street
New York, NY 10011

Export Sales to all countries except Canada,
France and French-speaking Switzerland:
Thames & Hudson
181A High Holborn Ltd.
London WC1V 7QX
England

Canadian Distribution:
Canadian Manda Group
One Atlantic Avenue, Suite 105
Toronto, Ontario M6K 3E7
Canada

Library of Congress Cataloging-in-Publication Data
Friedman, Lise.
    Alvin Ailey Dance Moves: a new way to exercise/ by Lise Friedman
        p. cm.
    ISBN 1-58479-285-X
        1. Dance. 2. Movement Education. 3. Exercise. 4. Ailey, Alvin. I. Title

GV1595.F75 2003
792.8—dc21

2003042449

Dance-and movement-based exercises are relatively risk-free, and should present
no health risk of any sort to most individuals. However, as with every form of
physical activity, if you live with, or suspect, a medical condition that may be
adversely affected by exercise such as heart disease, high blood pressure,
pregnancy, or other health issue, please consult your physician before undertaking
any of the exercises in this book.

The text of this book was composed in The Sans
Designed by Galen Smith and Priscilla Duty

Acknowledgments

A project of this scope could not have happened without many generous participants. A million thank-yous to all.

To the dancers, who generously gave their time and energy: Renee Robinson and Matthew Rushing, Alvin Ailey American Dance Theater; Kristina Michelle Bethel, Kirven J. Boyd, Robert Halley, Katherine Horrigan, Holly Alexis Hyman, Zach L. Ingram, Willy Laury, and Brandye Lee, Ailey II; Courtney Corbin, Julie Fiorenza, and James Pierce, B.F.A. program; and Steven McMahon, Certificate Program.

To the members of the Ailey organization, each one a crucial link in this process: Judith Jamison, Artistic Director, Alvin Ailey American Dance Theater; Denise Jefferson, Director, The Ailey School, and a welcoming and enthusiastic collaborator; Sylvia Waters, Artistic Director, Ailey II; Sharon Gersten Luckman, Executive Director, Alvin Ailey Dance Foundation; Jodi Krizer, Director of Marketing; Lynette Rizzo, Marketing Manager; Beth Olsen, Public Relations Manager; Ana Marie Forsythe, Chair, Horton Program and B.F.A. program Codirector; Tracy Inman, Codirector, Junior Division; Derrick W. Minter, Rehearsal Director, Ailey II; and Jon Taylor, Wardrobe Supervisor, Alvin Ailey American Dance Theater. Thank you to Nicholas Vergoth, for helping to pave the way.

To my unflappable and insightful editor Anne Kostick; photographer Chris Callis, for his way with light and form; designer Galen Smith, who with assistance from Priscilla Duty, made movement come alive on the page, and publisher Leslie Stoker, for her wholehearted embrace of this project.

Special thanks to my sister Ceil Friedman, a veteran of the aerobic wars, and friend and former dancer Megan Meade, for their willingness to test the exercises and advise as to what worked and what didn't. To my agent, Wendy Sherman, for her guidance, tenacity, and sense of humor. And to Margo Jefferson, for encouraging me to make the first phone call.

—Lise Friedman

Contents

Foreword

WELCOME TO THE WORLD OF ALVIN AILEY.

In 1970, when Alvin Ailey and Pearl Lang co-founded the Alvin Ailey American Dance Center in a spacious old church building on Manhattan's East 59th Street, they shared a philosophy about training the total dancer that was unusual for the times. Back then, ballet students were taught only ballet technique at such schools as the School of American Ballet, the American Ballet Theatre School, Ballet Arts, or the Dance Theatre of Harlem School. Students of modern dance studied at single-technique schools founded by dance pioneers like Merce Cunningham, Martha Graham, and José Limón. Mr. Ailey and Ms. Lang wanted extremely versatile dancers for their respective dance companies—those with flexibility in the upper torso, a sharpness of movement, and clear line of the legs. In order to do this they developed the school's broad curriculum, which included nine major dance techniques, cultural dance, classes to tone and strengthen the body, dance history, composition, and repertory.

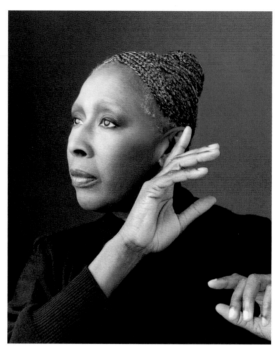

ARTISTIC DIRECTOR JUDITH JAMISON

When I was rehearsing at the Alvin Ailey American Dance Center (now known as The Ailey School), the energy was palpable. Students were eager to become accomplished in a variety of techniques—Horton, ballet, Graham-based modern, jazz, and of course, the technique of Katherine Dunham, an icon of modern dance. They gave their utmost in pursuit of that goal. This approach to dance training was visionary then. Maintaining this tradition at The Ailey School is an important and necessary way to prepare our students for the twenty-first century.

Each dance technique class (including the cultural dance of West Africa, Latin America the Caribbean, Spain and India) and somatic class (body conditioning, barre à terre and yoga) offered by our school trains your body in a contrasting, yet complementary manner. Different muscles are stretched and used in many ways. Your mind is also challenged to balance several different movement concepts at once. The result is that your body, your instrument, becomes capable of a larger expressive vocabulary, guided by a mind that embraces all ways of moving and a spirit that appreciates and enjoys the possibilities.

Alvin Ailey Dance Moves! offers you the chance to explore a wealth of experiences. The author, Lise Friedman, has done an insightful and meticulous job of selecting movement gems from many of the techniques and dance forms taught at our School. She has also interviewed our models for this book, in particular two Alvin Ailey American Dance Theater company members, the beloved Renee Robinson and the extraordinary Matthew Rushing, and has shared their anecdotes and insights about dance and dance life with you. In addition to Ms. Robinson and Mr. Rushing, eight dancers from Ailey II and four students from The Ailey School are featured throughout the book.

The creation of this book has truly been an act of community, mirroring the Ailey family. Many people have given generously of their time and expertise to bring this book to fruition including dancers from AAADT and Ailey II; students from The Ailey School; Sylvia Waters, Artistic Director of Ailey II; Denise Jefferson, Director of The Ailey School, and faculty members Ana Marie Forsythe, Celia Marino and Tracy Inman; and the Company's Executive Director, Sharon Gersten Luckman. Thanks to all of them.

—Judith Jamison
Artistic Director, Alvin Ailey American Dance Theater

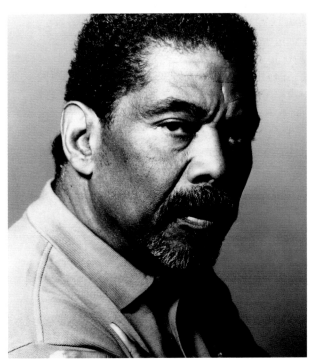

COMPANY FOUNDER ALVIN AILEY

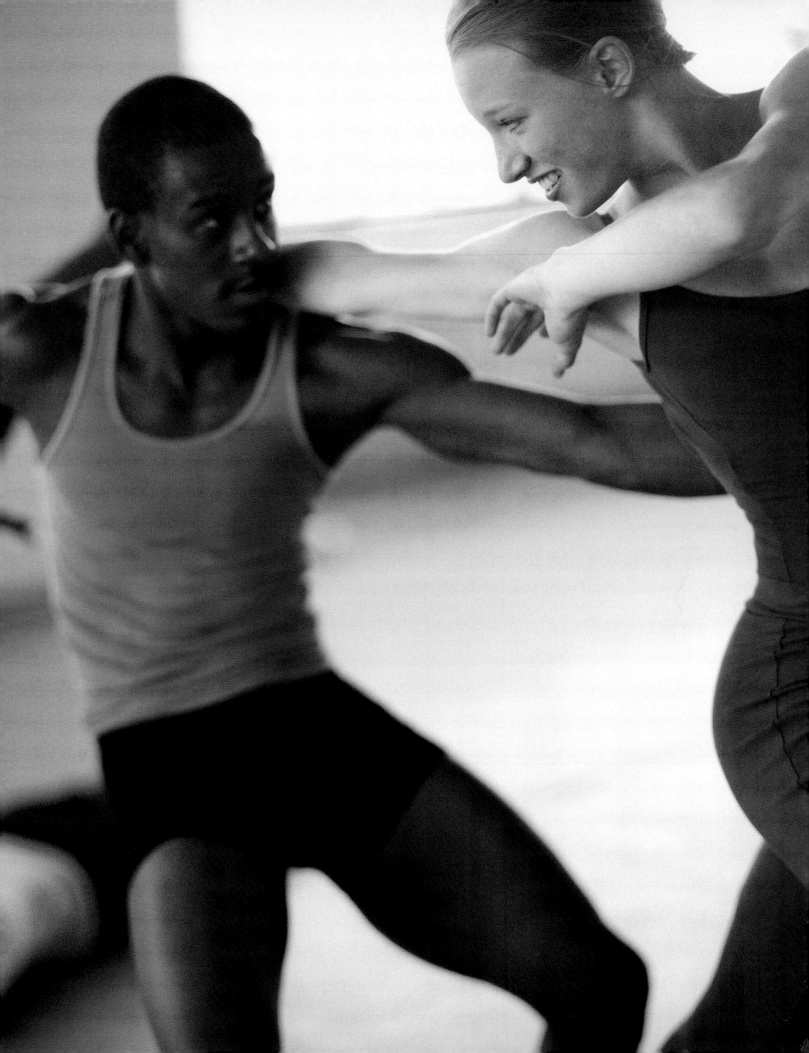

Introduction

When I started dance classes as a child, it never occurred to me that I was getting exercise along with the dancing. I was there for the sheer pleasure of moving through space, and captivated by the sense of fantasy my clever teachers encouraged in their young charges.

We didn't simply lift our arms overhead: We touched the stars with our fingertips, and in the process, lengthened our upper bodies. We never merely jumped: We vaulted treacherous "rivers," their banks defined by two ballet slippers placed just far enough apart to inspire a limb-stretching leap. Every image, no matter how whimsical, served our dancing and enhanced our physical development.

It wasn't too long before these fantasies gave way to more corporeal realities. I became hyperaware of what I could and couldn't do. My legs could fly way up, but I lost my bearings when I turned. Moving slowly and silkily felt divine, but rapid footwork tied my feet in a knot. I realized that desire was just a small component of what it would take to become a dancer.

This realization was accompanied by an understanding that every movement—from the most prosaic to the most exalted—had a profound effect on the body's shape, strength, and flexibility. And that the heightened self-awareness and physical well-being—that unmistakable endorphin-induced afterglow—that followed every class came from exerting myself fully, in an organized and directed fashion. I began to give dance its due as exercise.

I discovered that a careful warm-up not only prepared my muscles and joints for the rigorous movements to follow, it focused my mind and energy and ultimately freed me to concentrate on the dancing. I started to pay close attention to how a relatively simple movement like a demi plié—a small knee bend with heels rooted to the floor—simultaneously strengthens, stretches, and tones as it actively engages the buttocks, pelvis, inner thighs, and ankles.

Moving beyond the mechanics, I began to tap into the intention that drives every movement, developing a dance-motivated consciousness. In demi plié, for example, as the knees bend, the energy in the body radiates up and out, creating a sensation of vitality and buoyancy.

While typical exercise programs may work your muscles, after you've gotten over the novelty of the latest regimen, boredom begins to take over. Dance, on the other hand, puts you directly in touch with the pleasure of moving. It may be the most organic form of exercise, an instinctual response to music, the physical expression of our most primal impulses. Dance is a uniquely holistic form of movement that uses the entire body while feeding our longing for an aesthetically rich experience.

Dance also has tremendous, continuous impact on the quality of your relaxation, breathing, and rhythm, each of which increases bodily awareness and sensitivity and contributes to a heightened sense of well-being and self-esteem. You certainly won't get that sort of payback from a couple of hand weights.

It wasn't until I became a professional dancer subject to the needs of a single choreographer that I understood how working day in and day out within a specific technique or choreographic style molds your muscles in a certain way. One dancer may notice that her arms, though able to carve gorgeous arcs in space, are underdeveloped compared to her legs and feet. Another may find that despite an enviable ability to deliver gasp-inducing pirouettes, she feels insecure when trying to master a sustained balance.

Such weaknesses send alert dancers in search of techniques and training to fill in the perceived gaps. A modern dancer may dash across town to ballet class, a ballet dancer to a jazz or modern studio. Both may seek refuge at a yoga class, and they might even bump into each other at the gym.

Until 1989, the year I first visited The Ailey School to interview the late Alvin Ailey, I had never encountered a dance school that embraced the idea of comprehensive training so completely. Unlike other schools, which often adhere to one stylistically narrow technique, Ailey students experience a range of disciplines that prepare their bodies and minds for a spectrum of choreographic demands.

As I walked through the halls that day, I couldn't resist poking my head into various studios. One class was deep into Lester Horton's fortification studies. Another explored West Africa's dazzling polyrhythms and elastic, low-slung pelvis. Just a few doors down, dancers were absorbed in the reverie of a ballet adagio. Jazz, classical Indian, and improvisation classes were also taking place—and that was just one day's schedule.

It was, and continues to be a pioneering approach to creating a fit and versatile body, and one that presents limitless possibilities for exercise. You'll find that the process of enhancing one's physical condition needn't be plodding or routine. On the contrary, the program that you are about to encounter raises exercise to the realm of creativity and introduces dance-based movement as a way of life.

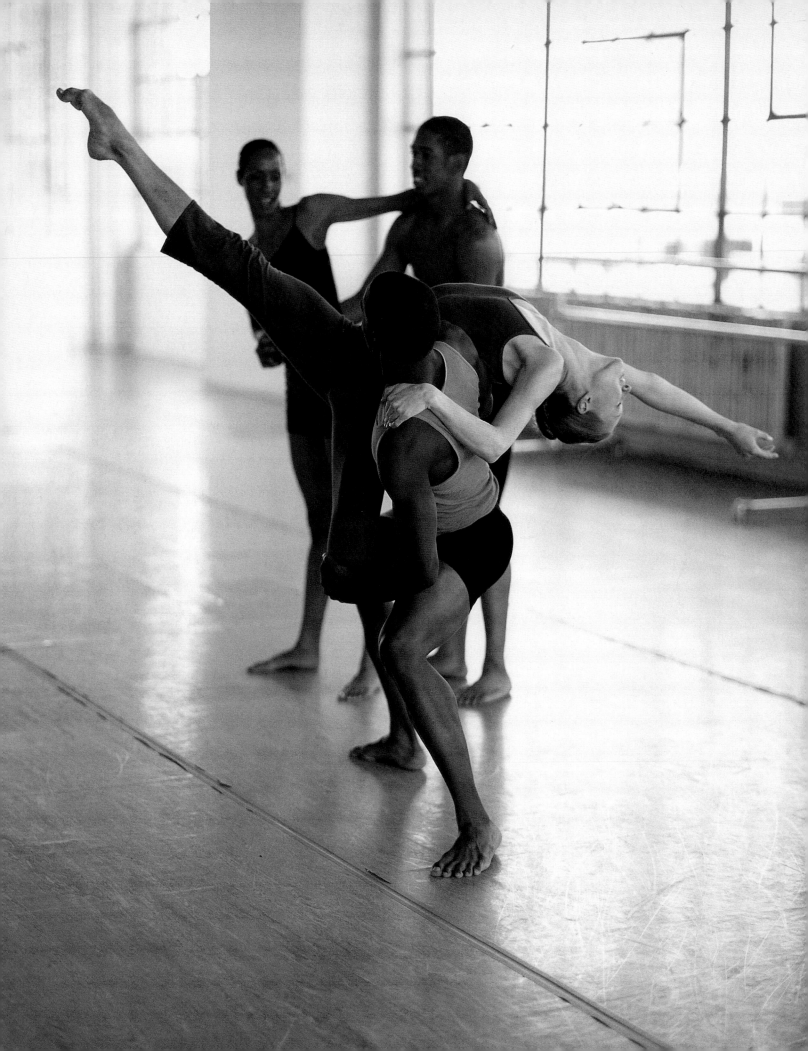

Where It All Comes From

The Alvin Ailey Approach to Movement

ROOTS AND INFLUENCES

If Alvin Ailey were here to tell us, he might say that his family's move from Rogers, Texas, to Los Angeles when he was twelve years old was the first significant event in a lifetime of artistic milestones. It was in Los Angeles, on a junior high school field trip to see a performance by the Ballet Russe de Monte Carlo, that Ailey had his initial encounter with the world of concert dance. That excursion, in turn, led to his exposure to the Afro-Caribbean aesthetic of the Katherine Dunham Dance Company, and eventually to another significant event, the beginning of Ailey's relationship with the pioneering choreographer Lester Horton.

It was Horton's enthusiastic embrace of ethnic cultures and his revolutionary mandate of inclusiveness that set him apart from his peers and so impressed the young Ailey. And then there was his supremely inventive modern dance technique. Upon Horton's death in 1953, Ailey assumed the directorship of his company and began creating his own dances. One year later, he and his close friend and fellow dancer Carmen de Lavallade appeared on Broadway in Truman Capote's *House of Flowers*.

New York City offered Ailey the opportunity to study with esteemed choreographers Doris Humphrey, Martha Graham, Hanya Holm, and Charles Weidman, among others, and to try his hand at acting as taught by Stella Adler. It was an intensely fertile period, rich with artistic influences and possibilities.

On March 30, 1958, at Manhattan's well-known 92nd Street Y, the curtain rose on the inaugural performance of Alvin Ailey American Dance Theater (AAADT). On that landmark program: Ailey's *Blues Suite,* a bittersweet homage to the boisterous Dew Drop Inn, a fixture of his Texas childhood. Made when Ailey was just twenty-seven years old, the dance revealed a choreographer blessed with an extraordinary ability to draw from and deftly combine a wealth of movement vocabularies into a potent whole. Signature movements from Horton technique, jazz, early twentieth-century social dances, and ballet all contribute to the dance's vivid language.

The company debut marked a singularly auspicious moment in dance history. Here was an artist with a uniquely expansive choreographic vision, one that would soon redefine the landscape of modern dance. Ailey's genius for translating his sense of what it meant to live in a dramatically changing America into luminous, culturally astute choreography not only altered the way audiences perceived dance; it forever altered their awareness of the African-American experience.

As American culture redefined itself, so did Ailey's ambitions for his company. What began as a small group of almost exclusively black dancers developed over the next few decades into an internationally revered, multi-ethnic repertory company of thirty-one dancers boasting a roster of nearly 200 works by more than seventy choreographers.

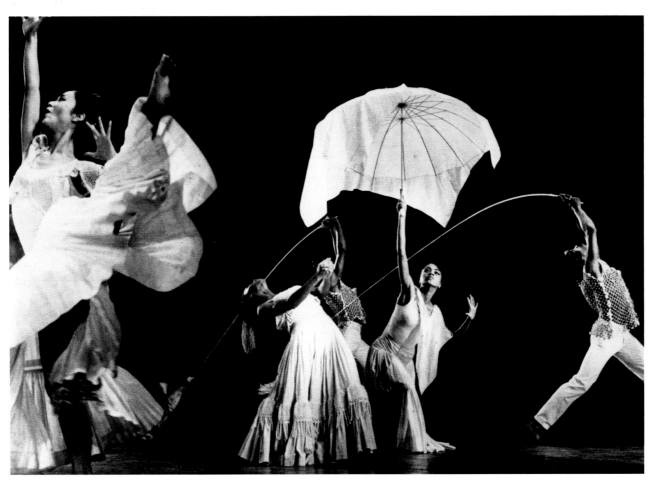

AN EARLY PERFORMANCE OF ALVIN AILEY'S SIGNATURE WORK, *REVELATIONS.*

In 1970 Ailey, with fellow choreographer Pearl Lang, started a school—a natural next step for an artist committed to giving everyone the chance to study dance. His edict: Dance classes will be open to the public. At the school's inception, there were 125 students enrolled. Today, under the expert direction of Denise Jefferson, upward of 3,500 dedicated dancers from around the world study at The Ailey School. Classes include everything from Horton, Dunham, and Graham-derived modern to ballet, jazz, classical Indian, and West African dance—even yoga, barre-à-terre, and body conditioning. Each class is an affirmation of Ailey's commitment to creating what he called "a whole spectrum of experience for the dancer as well as the audience."

That same line of thinking inspired the formation of the Alvin Ailey Repertory Ensemble, a workshop for exceptionally talented young dancers. Former Ailey dancer Sylvia Waters has served as artistic director since its inception in 1974. Now a professional company known as Ailey II, the twelve-member troupe nurtures future AAADT dancers and travels widely, a tireless ambassador of dance. In the last year alone, Ailey II dancers performed in forty-four U.S. cities, where, in addition to leading dozens of master classes and lecture-demonstrations, they gave more than sixty performances.

At the helm of all of this activity is Judith Jamison, a long-time star performer with AAADT, on Broadway, and with a number of companies around the world, as well as a choreographer. Jamison assumed the artistic directorship of Alvin Ailey American Dance Theater in 1989, shortly after Ailey's death and in accordance with his wishes. Under her stewardship, the Alvin Ailey Dance Foundation (AADF) has become a creative powerhouse that anticipates the artistic needs and desires of an increasingly global dance community.

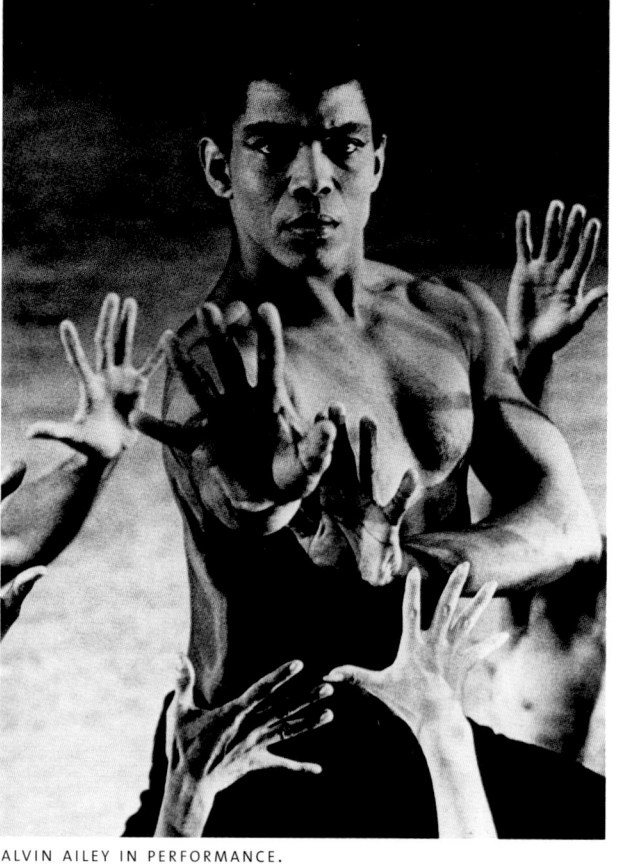

ALVIN AILEY IN PERFORMANCE.

In fall 2004, AADF will move into its new home, now under construction on the northwest corner of Fifty-fifth Street and Ninth Avenue in Manhattan. The building will be the country's largest structure dedicated to dance, encompassing an astonishing 77,000 square feet, twice the footage of the company's current space.

Within its walls will be a 5000-square-foot "black box" theater, a costume shop, a boutique, archive and library, and areas for physical therapy. Perhaps most expressive of Ailey's commitment to dance in its myriad manifestations: Twelve studios filled with dancers from the AAADT and AILEY II rehearsing and students discovering and progressing— exulting in Ailey's belief that "dance came from the people, and should always be delivered back to the people." If Alvin Ailey were here to tell us, he might say that this latest milestone is, indeed, a most significant event.

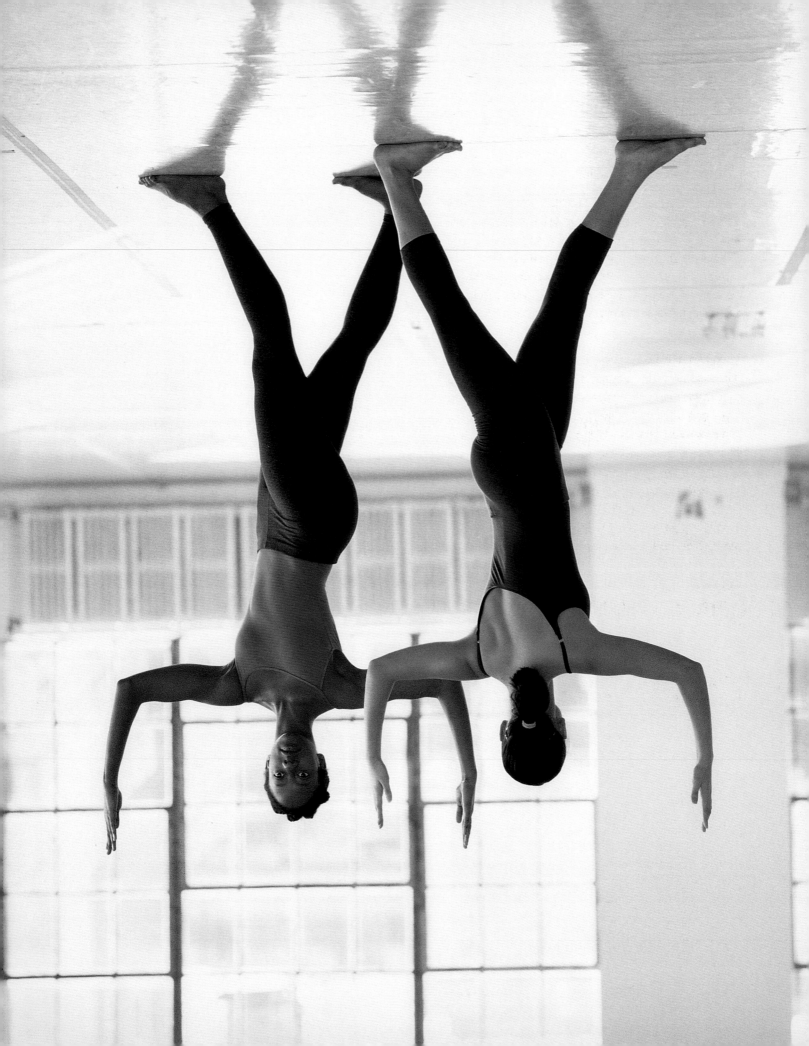

words of wisdom

You might be curious about what makes dancers tick; what inspires, motivates, challenges, and rewards them; how they form and maintain good habits, stay focused, and cope with fatigue and sore muscles; and what they do to carve out precious moments of quiet—of stillness—in the midst of a frenetic day. You'll find out all of this, and more, through the words of wisdom sprinkled throughout the book.

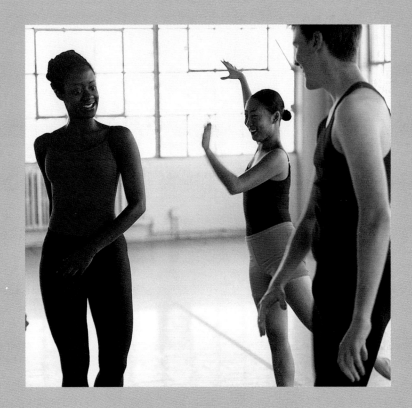

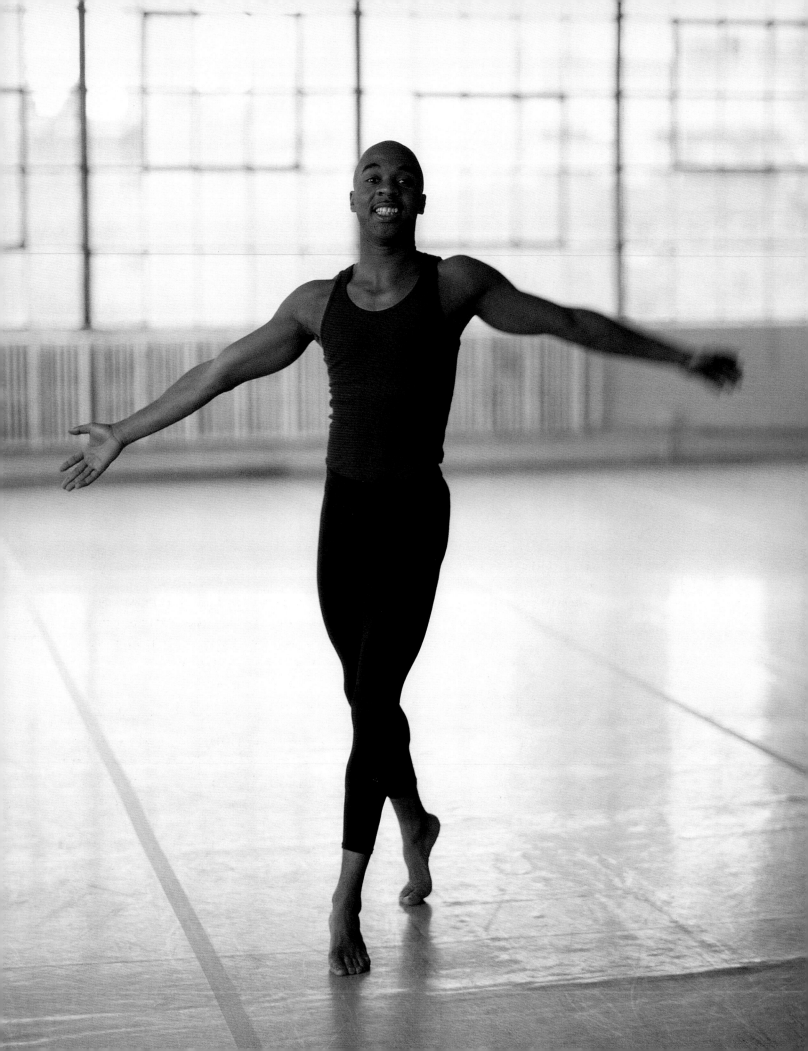

Techniques and Disciplines

The Ailey School's Eclectic Approach

Many of us look at dance with the avidity of birdwatchers, eager to identify and classify the style and origin of each and every movement. This is no small task, given that dance today is a multicultural feast of international influences: Jazz, tap, West African, Indian, Chinese, folk, swing, ballroom, flamenco, modern, postmodern, the tango, capoeira, ballet, kung-fu, and hip-hop are just a few of the forms that contribute to the inspiring kinetic mix. But it can be done. Just as every species of bird comes with a distinctive shape, markings, and song, there are signature qualities that distinguish each and every dance tradition and technique.

Dance or movement technique might be loosely defined as the most efficient way to execute a given physical task. But technique is a lot more than steps. It is a distinctive look—a particular attitude and method of getting from here to there—and it is usually grounded in specific exercises that have been developed to train the body to best fulfill the needs of the chosen material.

HORTON'S FORTIFICATION EXERCISES INSPIRED THIS MOVEMENT, PART OF AN EXERCISE ON PAGE **120**.

In dance parlance, "good technique" at its most basic means an awareness and mastery of the mechanics, including:

- proper alignment and placement of body parts
- strong, flexible, and responsive muscles
- the ability to execute a given movement

In addition to expertly conditioning and training your body, a comprehensive dance or movement technique should do the following:

- enhance your awareness of how your body moves, on its own and in tandem or counterpoint to other bodies
- teach you how to control and direct your energy
- increase your sensitivity to space and rhythm

Once these goals are achieved and the technique appears more or less effortless, it is then possible to inflect whatever movement you are doing with character and nuance; to move beyond mere mechanics into the realm of artistry.

The various techniques and movement styles taught at The Ailey School represent an unusually broad range of influences and traditions. It's the dance equivalent of cross-training. This is a direct reflection of Alvin Ailey and Judith Jamison's dedication to translating the human experience into dance, a multipronged approach that uses the body to its fullest while simultaneously developing versatile artists at home in any number of styles.

The pioneering techniques of Lester Horton and Katherine Dunham, as well as exercises based on that of Martha Graham, form the core of The Ailey School's modern dance curriculum. While all three evolved during the first half of the twentieth century and have in common the inventive shapes and dynamic rhythms that mark major modern dance techniques, each also emphasizes unique movement and spatial qualities.

Horton's fluid use of the limbs in counterpoint to a majestic, often cantilevering torso gives his technique striking elegance and force. Horton exercises are organized into an ingenious series of mini-dances he called "movement studies." These address choreographic concepts such as changing levels, rhythmic impetus, shape, weight, volume, and tempo while stretching, strengthening, and sensitizing the entire body. The Horton-trained dancer is at ease, whether teetering magnificently on half-toe or plunging headfirst into a deep, hinging fall.

Graham's principles of spinal contraction and release and the angular rigor of her movements create a powerful and organic connection to the solar plexus and to the floor. Like all modern dance techniques, Graham's technique developed over decades along with and in service to the choreography. The result is an eminently logical syllabus of strengthening and stretching exercises that both underscore and amplify the body's innate capabilities. A class typically starts on the floor; progresses to standing extensions, balances, and falls; and culminates in exercises that travel across the floor.

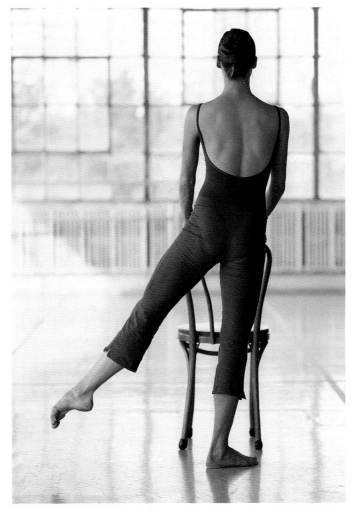

THIS VARIATION, FROM BALLET'S BARRE EXERCISES, IS IN THE STRENGTH CHAPTER ON PAGE 140.

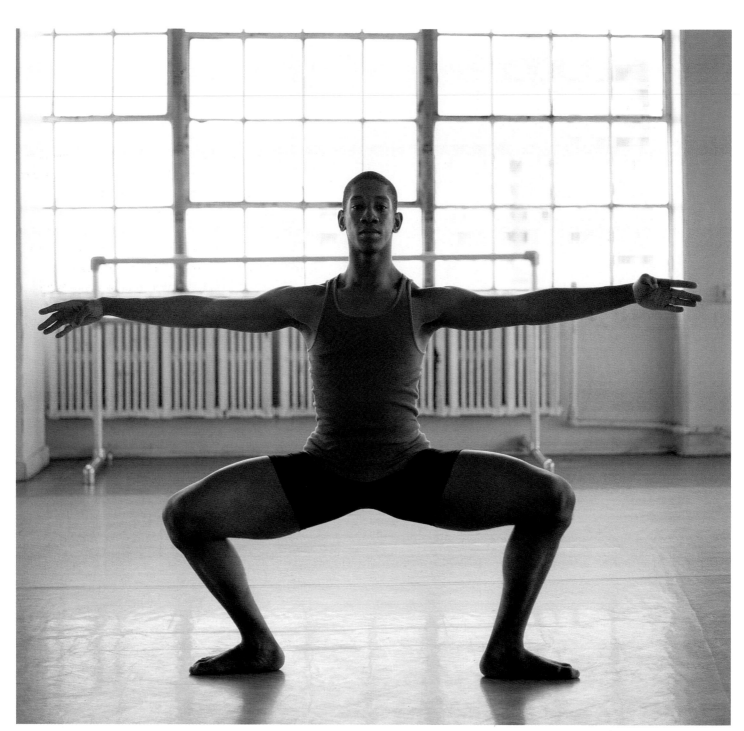

ONE ASPECT OF SOME WEST AFRICAN DANCE IS A LOW-SLUNG PELVIS, AS IN THIS EXERCISE ON PAGE 160

Dunham technique combines the undulating torso, isolated limbs, and unrestrained pelvis that characterize African and Caribbean dance styles with elements of ballet and other modern dance forms.

Ailey students also learn the jutting isolations and dynamism of jazz, West African dance's driving rhythms and graceful curving arms, and the extended line and lyricism of ballet, a technique that supports virtually every other through its concentration on form—how a shape or movement is executed. Further physical refinement comes from classical Indian dance's filigreed arms and hands and intricate rhythms, yoga's superlative integration of body and mind, and the targeted strengthening and stretching of body conditioning.

The exercises and movement studies featured in this book draw from many of these techniques. The Warm-up chapter, for example, includes exercises adapted from yoga, Horton, and jazz. The stretching exercises are culled from body conditioning and classical Indian dance, among other disciplines. Each exercise emphasizes the technique—the "how-to" that enables you to execute the movement correctly and efficiently—as well as the accompanying artistic components that make dance-based exercise and movement both a physically pleasurable and aesthetically pleasing experience.

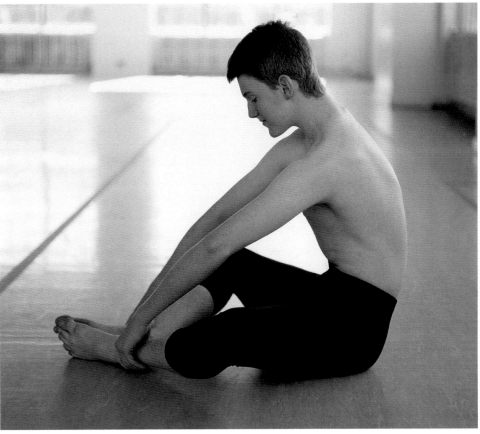

THE SPINAL CONTRACTION SEEN IN MARTHA GRAHAM'S DANCE TECHNIQUE INSPIRED THIS MOVEMENT ON PAGE 74.

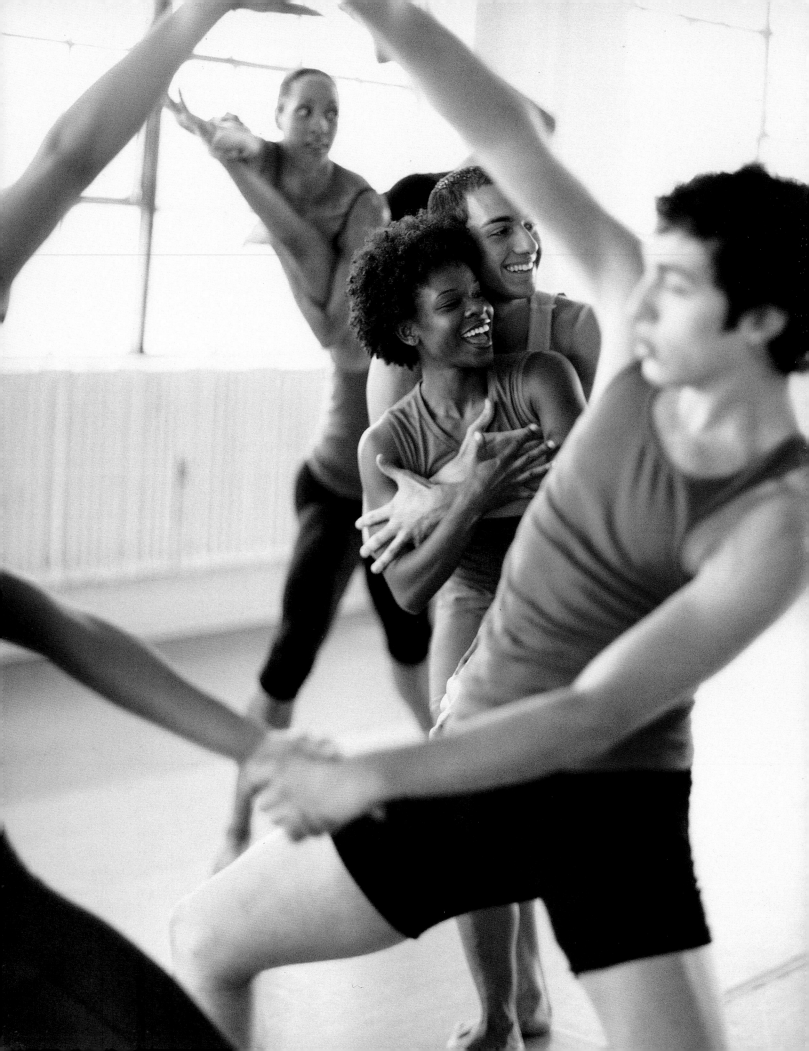

Putting this Book to Work

The fact that you have *Alvin Ailey Dance Moves!* in your hands is proof positive of your love of dance—and of your enthusiasm and eagerness to get in shape. The challenging part is allowing yourself the time to gain flexibility and strength. You may already have a certain amount of both, but you want to be sure to start slowly and work carefully and consistently.

Every well-designed exercise program emphasizes individual achievement—and this one is no exception. Remember to work toward your personal best rather than pushing for unattainable results that could cause injury. Your own fitness goals are what count, and it's your commitment to those goals that will yield tangible results.

It is important to keep in mind that because dancers spend most of their time working with their bodies—and have been doing so for years—they have a leg up on the rest of us. Rome wasn't built in a day and neither are our muscles. Take pleasure and care in the execution of these exercises, and your progress will follow.

You are no doubt wondering how frequently you should work out. Like dancers everywhere, the Ailey-trained dancers featured in these pages attend daily dance classes and log considerably many more movement hours during rehearsals and performances. So it follows that the more often you exercise, within reason of course, the more quickly you will feel and see results.

But, unlike professional dancers, your life is probably filled with activities that are unrelated to continuous movement. The solution: Fit your workout into whatever time you do have. If you can manage a daily exercise routine, that's great (see page 28-30 for various options). If not, try to carve out some time every other day or even three times a week. Pick a schedule that works for you, then make an effort to be consistent. One beauty of exercise is that it's fluid; you can always make adjustments.

Pay close attention to the step-by-step photographs of the dancers that accompany the written instructions. These expert demonstrations of the exercises should serve as your guide and inspiration. Try to "listen" to your body as you do the exercises. Some movements will feel more comfortable than others. You also may find that certain parts of your body are strong but not flexible and vice versa; this is perfectly normal. Your objective is to eventually strike a healthy balance between the two.

If a position or movement feels odd or uncomfortable, take a moment to check the photographs and instructions to be sure you're executing the movement correctly. You may need to adjust your technique—*how* you do the exercise— or perhaps you simply need time to become accustomed to something new.

On the other hand, if something hurts, stop immediately! None of these exercises should cause you pain, much less injury, but you may have a weakness or vulnerability that makes some of these movements painful. Use your judgment. It may make sense to try again tomorrow. If the pain is sharp or severe, you should consult your physician. You're trying to achieve a sense of inner harmony along with improved fitness, which is not possible if you hurt.

Essentials

If all you can manage is 7–10 minutes, do this essential sequence. You'll feel better for it and won't lose your workout momentum.

WARM-UP

Bend and Breathe   PAGE 35

Roll Down   PAGE 38

Knees to Chest   PAGE 40

Shoulder Rolls   PAGE 46

Neck Warmer   PAGE 48

STRETCH

Calf Stretch   PAGE 102

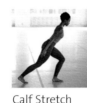

Handiwork   PAGE 108

STRENGTH

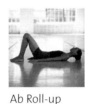

Ab Roll-up   PAGE 114

Here is an abbreviated series of exercises from all six chapters for the days when you have just 20–30 minutes to spare.

STRENGTH

Ab Roll-up   PAGE 114

Incline Push-up   PAGE 124

Heel Slide   PAGE 126

Demi Plié   PAGE 136

Press and Flick   PAGE 138

BALANCE AND COORDINATION

The Dancer   PAGE 148

Do The Pony   PAGE 156

RELAXATION AND REJUVENATION

Loosen Up   PAGE 182

Face Time   PAGE 184

Constructive Rest   PAGE 194

The Shortcut Program

WARM-UP

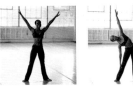

Bend and Breathe   PAGE 36

Roll Down   PAGE 38

Knees to Chest   PAGE 40

Shoulder Rolls   PAGE 44

Neck Warmer   PAGE 48

Forward Swing and Release PAGE 54

POSTURE AND ALIGNMENT

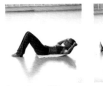

Lumbar Sling   PAGE 68

Basic Spinal Twist   PAGE 72

Port de Bras   PAGE 76

STRETCH

Hip Lift   PAGE 90

Hamstring Stretch   PAGE 92

Lunging Stretch   PAGE 100

Calf Stretch   PAGE 102

Handiwork   PAGE 106

The exercises in this book are organized into a complete, physically logical program. Each chapter focuses on a particular, essential component of your workout routine.

WARM-UP
Gentle exercises that wake up, invigorate, and prepare your body and mind for movement.

POSTURE AND ALIGNMENT
Floor, sitting, and standing exercises that enhance your posture awareness while helping to stretch, strengthen, and elongate your spine.

STRETCH
Carefully calibrated floor, sitting, and standing stretches that increase your joint and muscle flexibility as well as your range of movement.

STRENGTH
Effective exercises that progressively tone and shape your abdominals; upper, middle, and lower back; gluteals, hamstrings, quadriceps, calves, and feet; and your shoulders, arms, and hands.

BALANCE AND COORDINATION
Standing and moving exercises that center, orient, and propel you through space with grace and confidence.

RELAXATION AND REJUVENATION
Stretching, breathing, and relaxation exercises that help you decompress, release tension, and recharge your batteries.

If executed from start to finish, the exercises will take you between 60 and 90 minutes to complete. As you become accustomed to the routine and more physically adept, you may be able to complete it more quickly.

There will, of course, be days when your time is limited. The Shortcut Program (see page 28) is a streamlined version of the full program that touches all the bases and will take you about 20 to 30 minutes to complete.

For days so packed that you can devote just a few minutes to exercise, the seven-to-ten-minute Essentials (see page 30) sequence ensures that those precious moments are put to their best possible use. It's a great routine for anyone with a demanding travel schedule working out in a cramped hotel room.

If you wish to concentrate on a particular aspect of the exercise program (posture and alignment or strengthening exercises, for example) start with Essentials, then simply proceed with the exercises in your chapter of choice. As always, no matter how much or how little time you have, don't forget to stretch! (See Stretch, page 87, for much more about this most important activity.)

NOTE: The number of repetitions suggested for individual exercises is meant to serve as a guide. You may choose to do fewer repetitions or, as you make progress, increase the number of repetitions of a given exercise.

The Exercises

SETTING THE STAGE

A calm, comfortable environment, as free as possible of distractions, is a key component of a successful workout session. Check the list below for some essentials that will help you set up your environment to make the most of your routine.

- stretchy or loose clothing that allows you to move freely
- bare feet to allow your peds the full benefit of your workout and so that you won't slip
- a rug, mat, or towel to provide cushioning and warmth during floorwork
- a straight-back chair for seated exercises and, occasionally, for balance
- enough floor space to fully extend your limbs while lying down; if you can manage to find a space with some traveling room, all the better
- music that sets the mood (see The Music Made Me Do It! page 199)
- a bottle of still water to keep you hydrated during your workout. Be sure to drink a glass or two before you begin exercising and, of course, again when you finish.

READINESS

Before you begin these exercises, turn down the volume on your answering machine so you won't be tempted to answer the phone. And close the door. Tell anyone who might wander through your space, not to!

A NOTE ABOUT FOOD AND EXERCISE

There are no hard-and-fast rules, but you will feel most comfortable and enjoy a more efficient workout if you don't exercise on a full stomach. You should wait at least thirty minutes after eating a meal. If you've just consumed a gigantic meal, you should wait considerably longer. Of course, if you've just eaten a small, nutritious snack, you can get started as soon as you like.

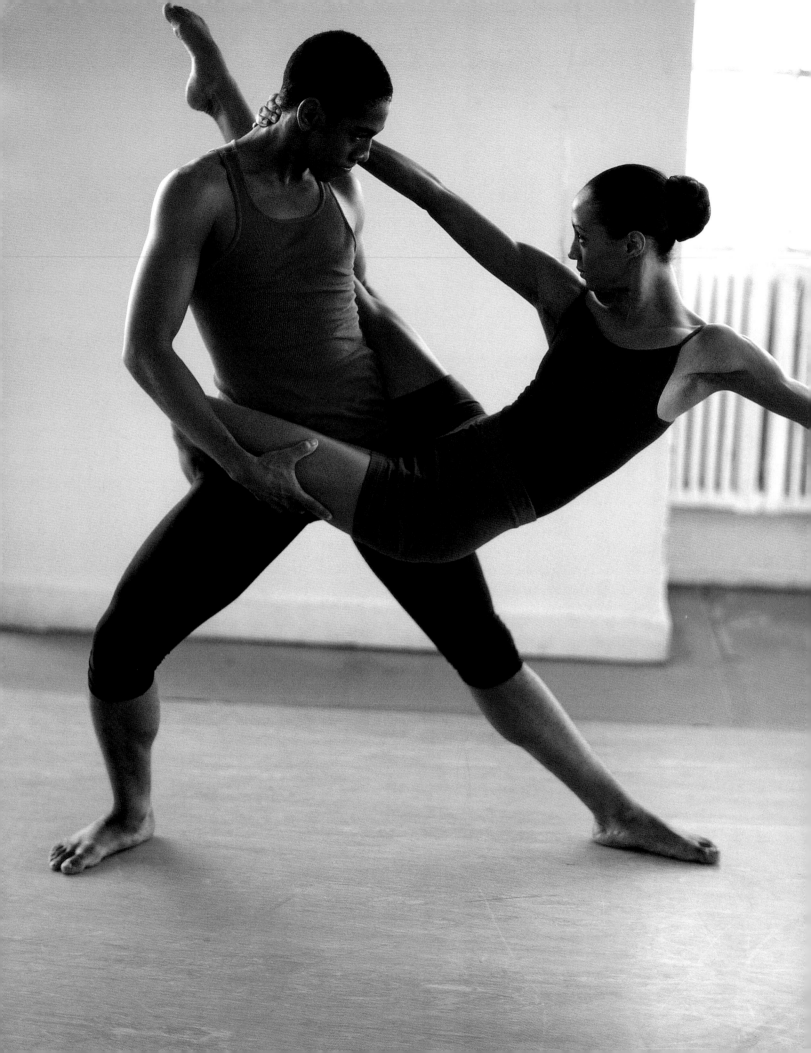

*Chicken
for
breakfast*

Warm-up

Every dance class—indeed, each and every well-designed exercise routine—should be preceded by a methodical and progressive warm-up. This essential first step gets your blood moving and warms, energizes, and coordinates your muscles so they can work together efficiently, without undue stress or strain. As its name suggests, a warm-up raises your internal, or core, temperature from its cooler resting state as it gently wakes up and invigorates your body, preparing it for movement.

Equally important, a warm-up helps focus your mental energy on the task at hand and readies your mind for the more demanding exercises to follow. The more concentrated and aware you are during each step of your warm-up, the more effective and safe your exercise routine will be.

Some dancers need to spend extra time warming up their hip joints; others may be more concerned about readying their backs. Every body is different. As you proceed through the warm-up exercises below, you will begin to get a sense of your own body's weaknesses and strengths—and to which areas you may wish to devote more or less effort.

Through these warm-up exercises, you will also begin to develop a keen appreciation for the energy and quality of your movement. Discovering how your body occupies and moves through space is, after all, a fundamental joy of dancing.

Bend and Breathe

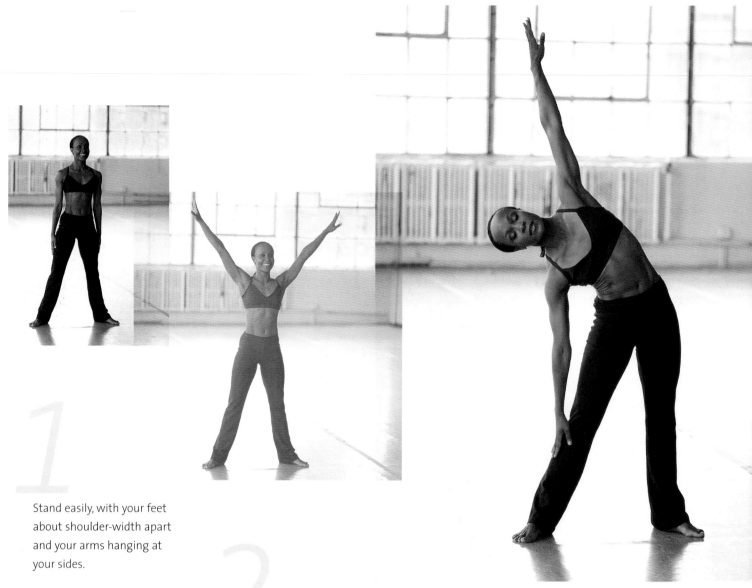

1

Stand easily, with your feet about shoulder-width apart and your arms hanging at your sides.

2

Inhale and slowly lift your arms out to your sides then over your head to form a wide V.

3

Exhale and tilt your torso to your right side, at the same time lowering your right arm until it touches your leg. Keep reaching out with your left arm; try to keep your hips still.

This exercise helps establish the rhythm of your breath as it wakes up your body. Move slowly and smoothly.

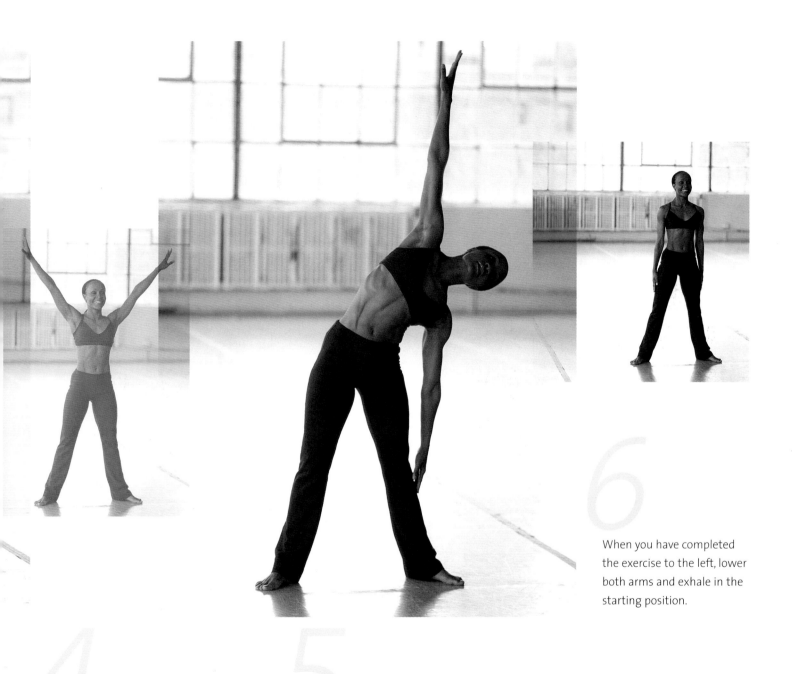

6

When you have completed the exercise to the left, lower both arms and exhale in the starting position.

4

Inhale as you lift your torso and raise both arms overhead again.

5

Repeat to your left side.

Repeat the bend-and-breathe cycle four times.

Roll Down

This exercise warms up and stretches your spine.

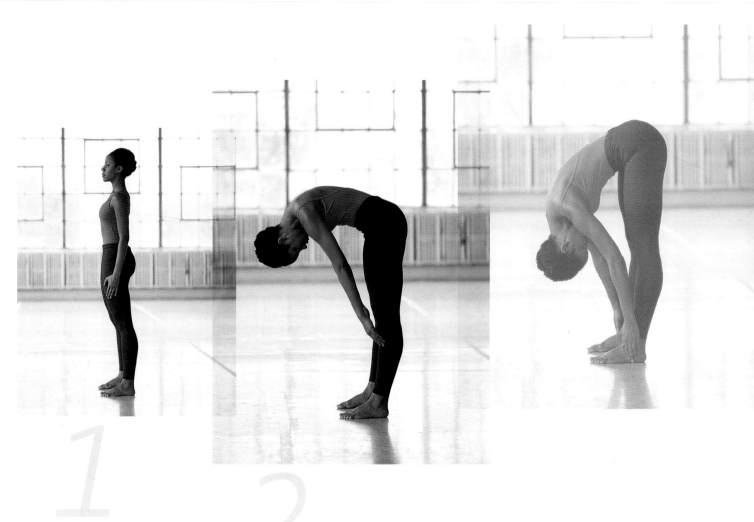

1

Stand with your feet parallel and your arms hanging comfortably at your sides. Inhale deeply.

2

Exhale and bend your knees slightly as you slowly drop your head, shoulders, upper back, and then your torso, until your head and hands hang toward the floor.

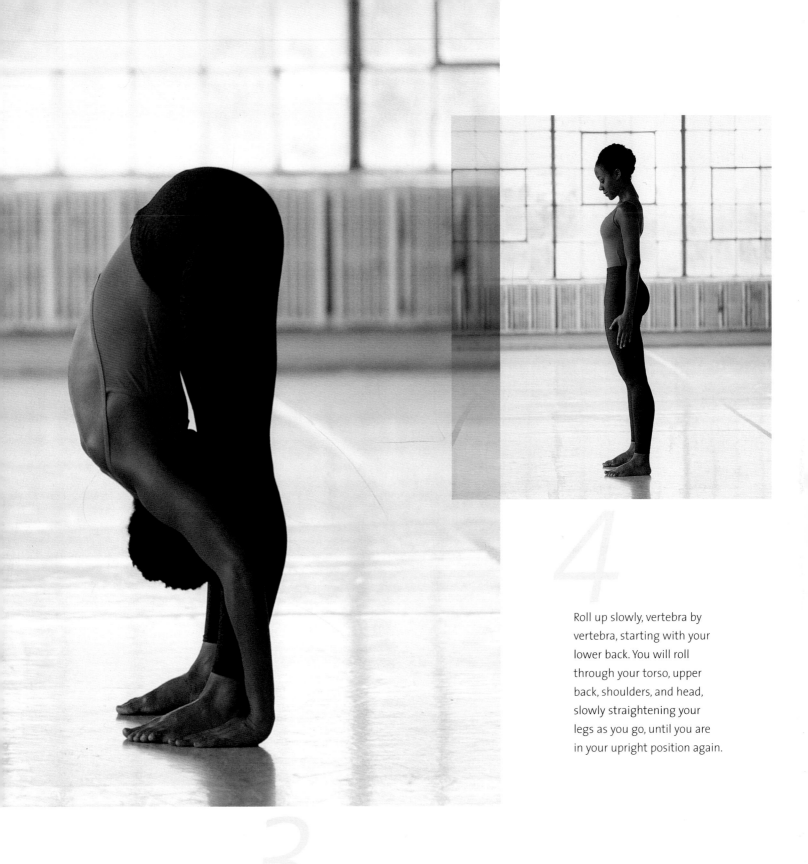

4

Roll up slowly, vertebra by vertebra, starting with your lower back. You will roll through your torso, upper back, shoulders, and head, slowly straightening your legs as you go, until you are in your upright position again.

3

If you have the flexibility, reach down even farther until your palms rest on the floor and your forehead touches your knees.

Repeat the roll down three or more times, breathing more deeply each time and working to increase your stretch.

Knees to Chest

This easy knee lift warms up your hip joints and gets your abdominals working.

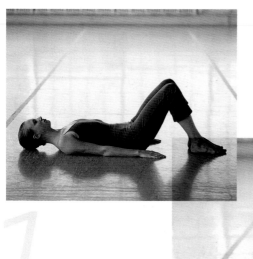

1

Lie on your back with your knees bent in parallel and the soles of your feet flat on the floor. Your arms should be extended, palms down, along the sides of your body.

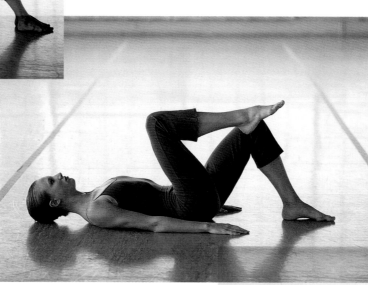

2

Lift your right knee toward your chest. As you lift, press your lower back into the floor, creating a concave semicircle with your abdomen. Try to keep both hips on the floor.

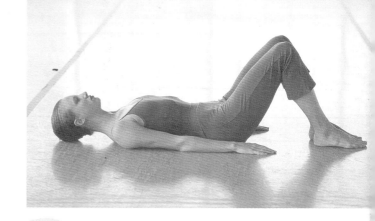

3

Lower your knee to the starting position.

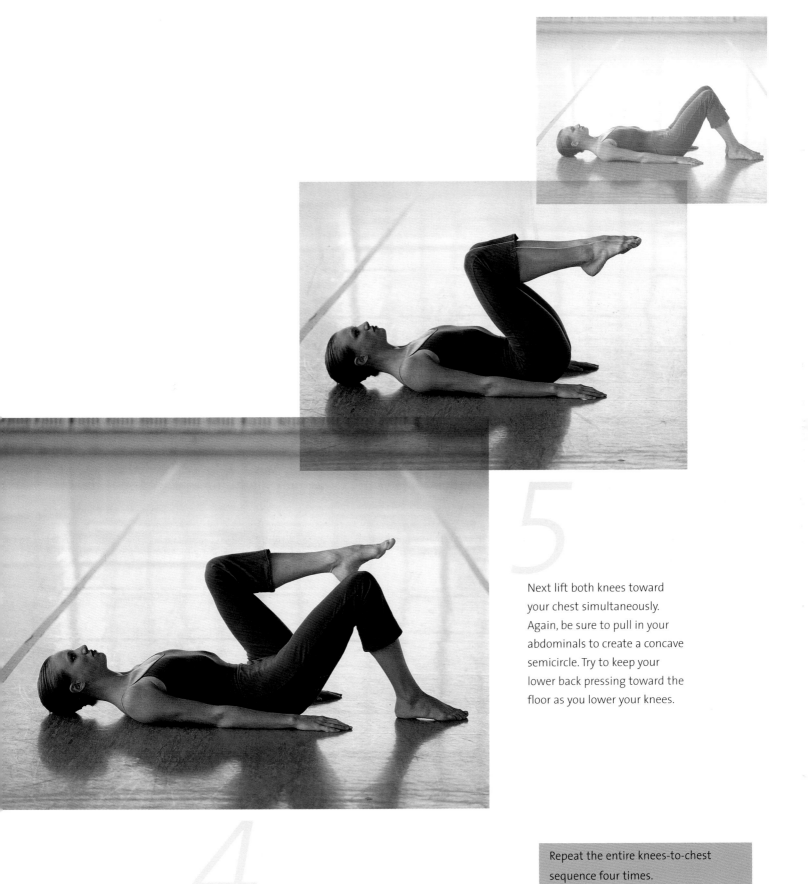

5

Next lift both knees toward your chest simultaneously. Again, be sure to pull in your abdominals to create a concave semicircle. Try to keep your lower back pressing toward the floor as you lower your knees.

Repeat the entire knees-to-chest sequence four times.

4

Repeat with your left leg.

Pretzel

This lower-back-warmer is a dancer's favorite. It may seem awkward at first, but after you try it a few times—and feel how good it makes your back feel—you'll be hooked.

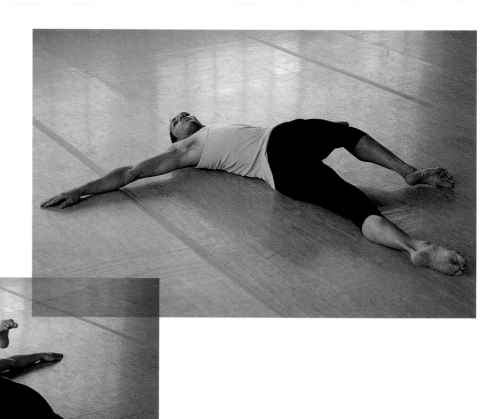

2 Lift your right knee toward your chest.

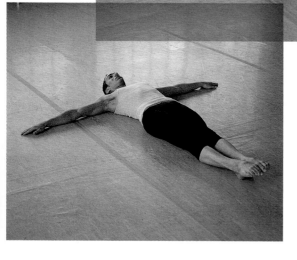

1 Lie on your back with your legs together, extending straight from your pelvis. Your arms should be stretched to form a T with your palms facing the floor.

3 Slowly lower your knee toward the floor so it falls below your left arm, breathing deeply and trying to relax into the twist. If your knee can't reach the floor, that's okay—you will still feel the stretch. Move your upper body and shoulders as little as possible. If your right shoulder lifts as you twist, counteract it by stretching your right arm further out along the floor.

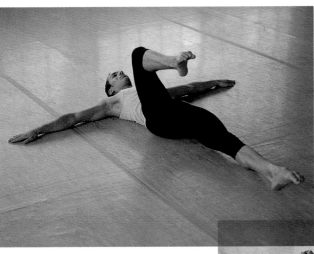

4 When you're ready, lift your right knee off the floor, returning it to your chest.

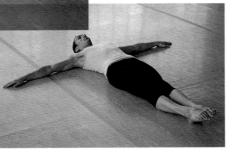

5 Lower your leg slowly until it is fully extended on the floor again.

Repeat the entire pretzel sequence with your left leg. Then alternate legs three or four more times.

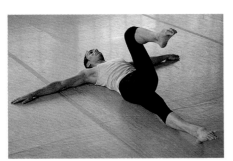
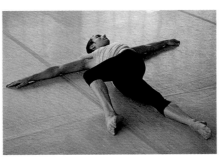
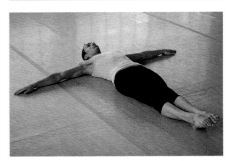

Shoulder Rolls

Prepare your shoulders for movement and release tension with this exercise, which may be done standing or seated.

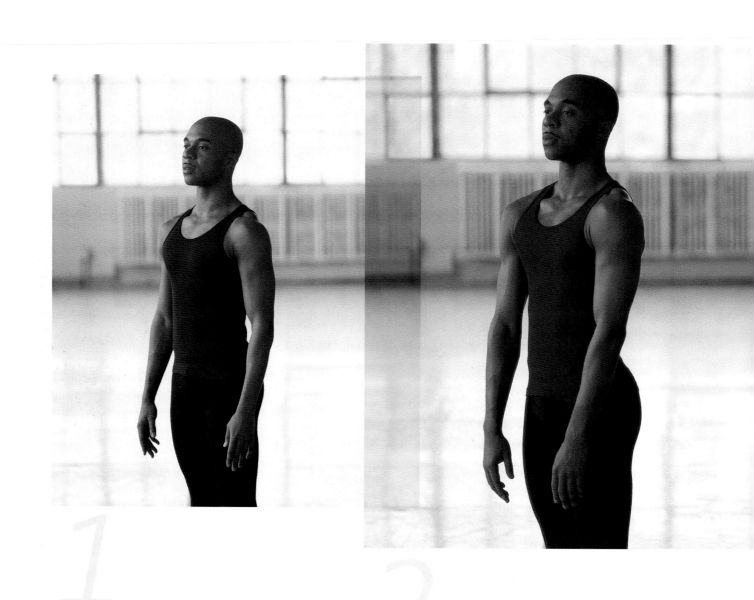

1

Stand or sit easily, with your arms hanging loosely at your sides.

2

Rotate your shoulders simultaneously in a smooth circle, moving them forward, up, back, and down. As you circle your shoulders, try to keep your torso quiet and your back long.

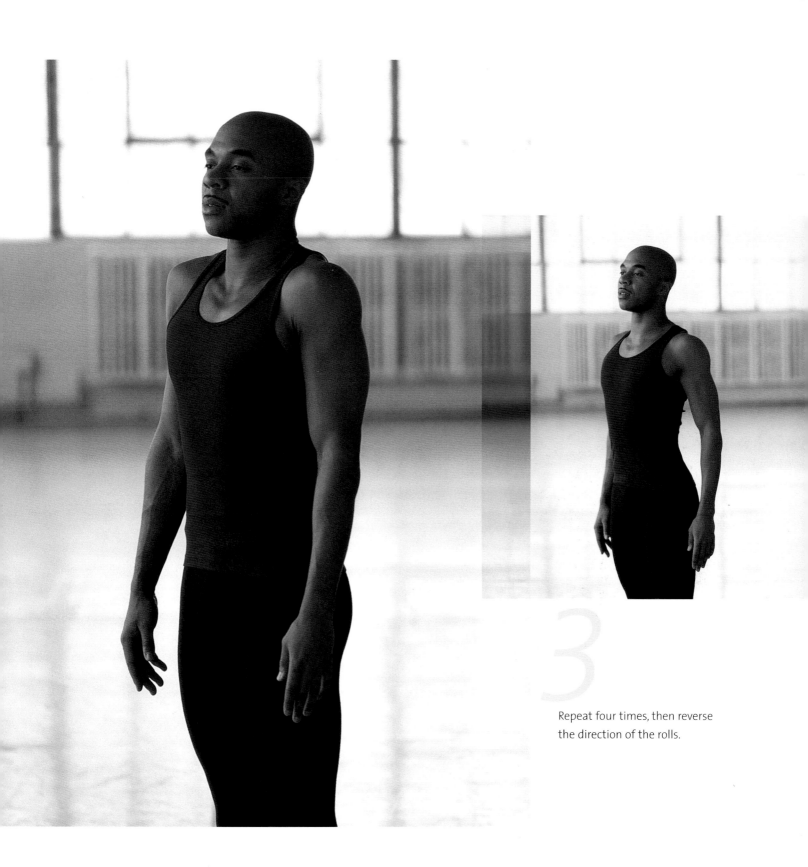

3

Repeat four times, then reverse
the direction of the rolls.

CONTINUED >

Shoulder Rolls

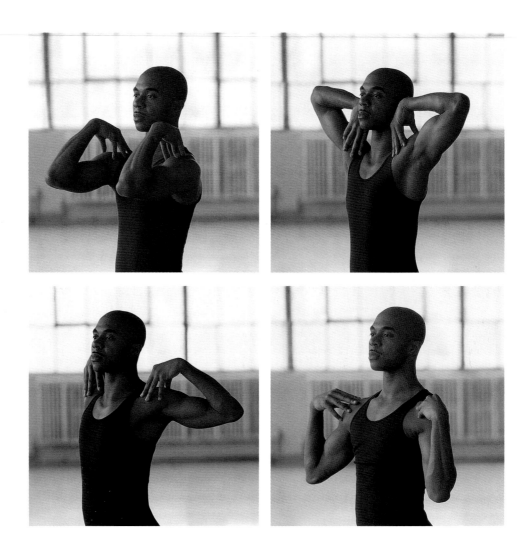

4

Next, place your hands on your shoulders—your elbows should be extended like wings—and repeat the circling action, first in one direction, then in the other. You should lead with your elbows.

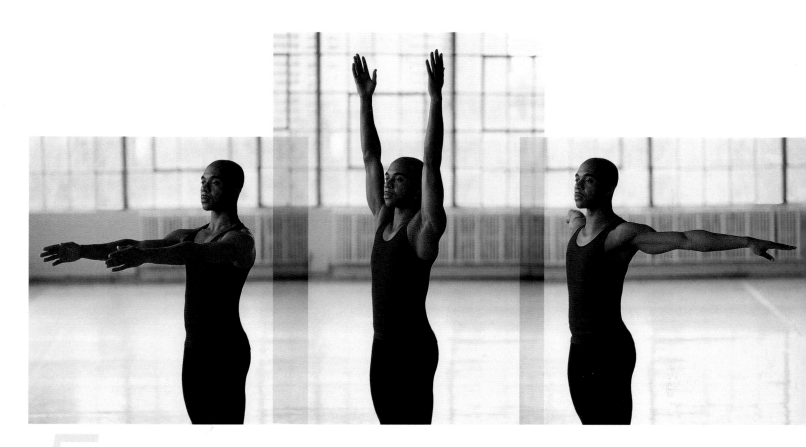

5

Now extend your arms fully and repeat the forward-and-back sequence in both directions. This time you should lead with your hands and fingers.

HINT When you reach to the back, be careful not to go so far that your chest and shoulders rise: make sure your upper torso is relaxed.

Neck Warmer

Your neck requires a gentle but focused warm-up.
Neck warmers may be done standing or seated.

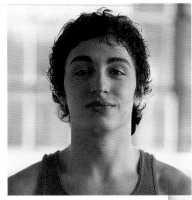

1

Begin with your head facing
forward. Your neck and back
should be long and your
shoulders relaxed.

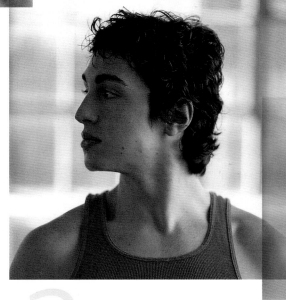

2

Turn your head to your right
as far as is comfortable. Try
to keep your shoulders facing
forward and your chin level as
you feel the stretch at the base
of your neck. Return your head
to the center.

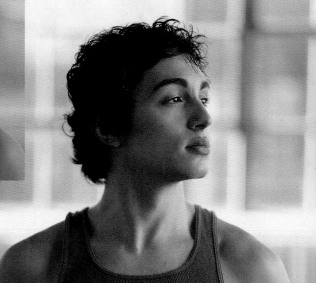

3

Turn your head to your left.
Then return to center.

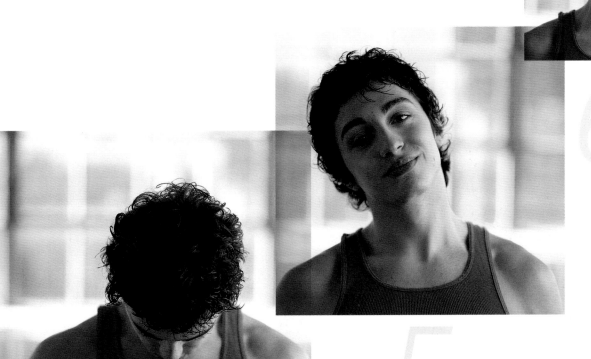

6

Return your head to the center and repeat, this time tilting your head toward your left shoulder.

5

Next, while keeping your head facing forward, tilt your right ear toward your right shoulder. Be aware of your left shoulder — do not allow it to hike up. You will feel the muscles working on both sides of your neck.

4

Now tilt your chin toward your chest. Feel the weight of your head and keep your shoulders relaxed. Return your head to center. Repeat the entire sequence — turning your head to the right, left, and down — three or four times.

Repeat this neck-warmer sequence four times.

Hip Pivot

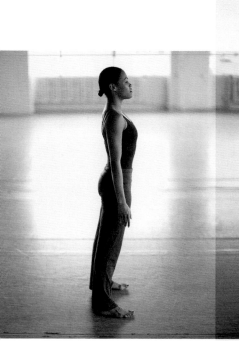

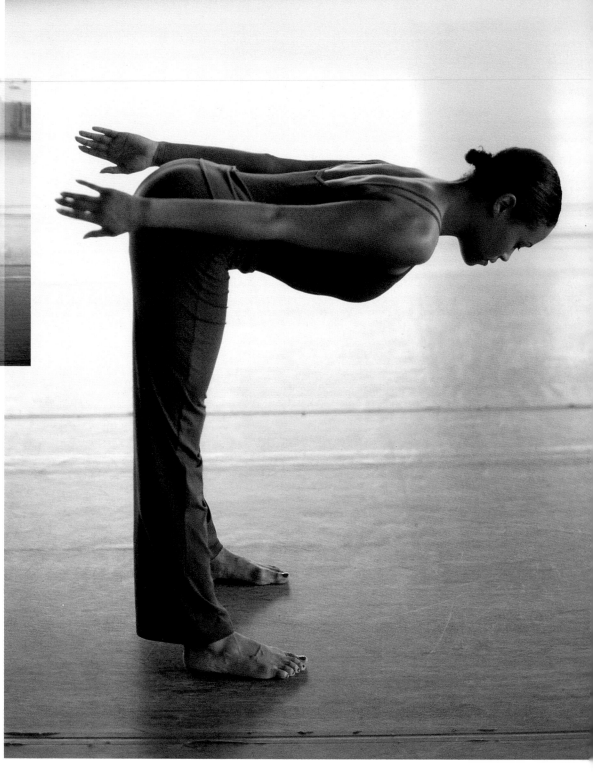

1

Stand upright, with your arms
hanging comfortably at your
sides and your legs in the
position choreographer Lester
Horton called "parallel second."
This means that your feet are
parallel to each other—toes
facing forward—and opened
to the width of your pelvis.

Warm up and stretch your calves, hamstrings, lower back, and abdominal muscles with this exercise.

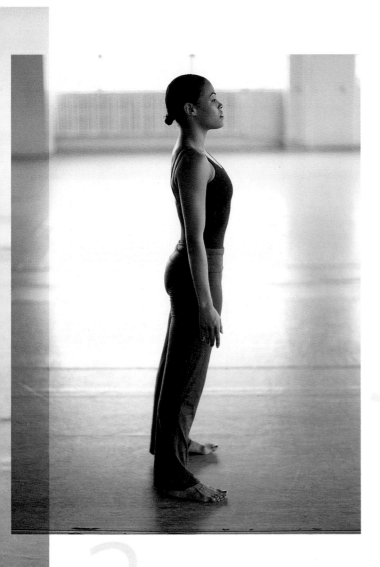

3

When you've bent as far as is comfortable while maintaining a long back, slowly lift your torso back to the upright position to a slow count of four. Feel the lift in your abdominal muscles.

2

Bend forward to a slow count of four, with a hinging action from your hip joint, keeping your back as flat as possible. Your goal is to eventually create a right angle at your hip joints. Your arms should stay at your sides; try to keep your kneecaps lifted and your neck long.

Repeat the hip pivot two or three times, each time bringing your awareness to the hinging action in your hips.

HINT As you do this exercise, try to keep your weight moving forward toward the balls of your feet, rather than allowing yourself to sink back onto your heels. Your energy should move forward and out.

Feet First

Because dancers are among the most feet-fraught among us, they are a great source for feet-fixing exercises. The supremely elegant appendages that we see onstage are in reality subject to a staggering range of abuses, including hours of pounding on unforgiving surfaces. Here's how dancers keep their toes supple.

1. Sit in a straight-back chair with both feet flat on the floor. Lift your right leg slightly off the floor, bending your knee a little bit more.

2. Keeping your calf as relaxed as possible, rotate your foot four times clockwise, then four times counterclockwise. Flex your toes at the top of the circle (when your toes point up) and point them at the bottom (when they point down). Feel the stretch in your instep, arch, and your Achilles tendon (the extremely strong tendon that connects your calf muscles to the bone of your heel).

3. Repeat the circles with your left foot.

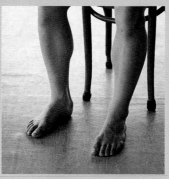
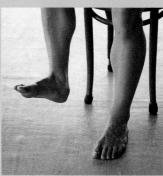
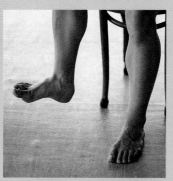
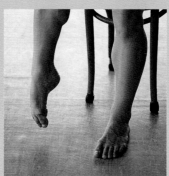
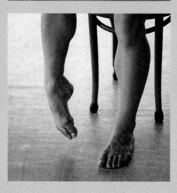

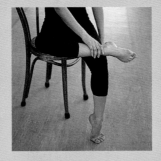

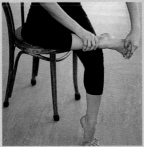

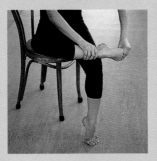

Massage

Self-massage is a great way to wake up your body. Your feet respond especially well to hands-on treatment. You'll find this exercise easiest to do while seated.

1. Place your right foot on top of your left thigh, allowing your right knee to open to the side.

2. Using your right hand to stabilize your ankle, massage your upper foot and toes with your left hand. Press your toes back toward your shin and press them forward toward your heel. Feel the stretch along the top and bottom of your foot.

3. Lace your fingers between your toes and squeeze them apart.

4. Massage your arch and instep with firm, smooth strokes. Use your thumb to apply as much pressure as is comfortable.

5. Move to your heel. Pay special attention to spots that feel especially tender. Be sure to rub the area where your Achilles tendon connects to your heel, at the back of your ankle.

6. Place your right foot gently on the floor and repeat the massage on your left foot.

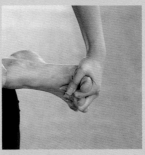

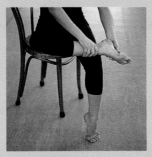

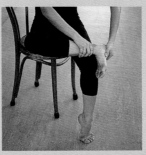

Forward Swing and Release

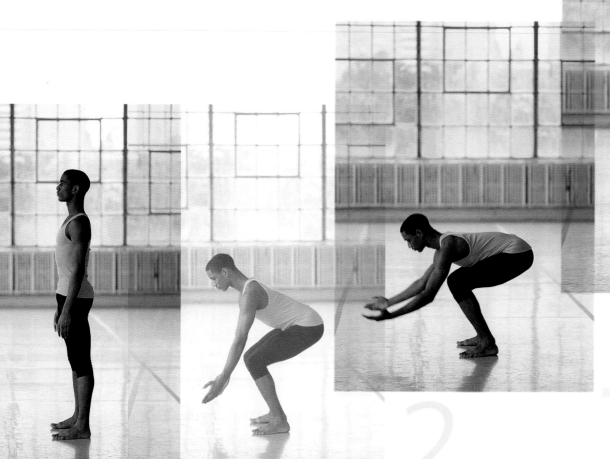

1
Stand with your feet parallel and about two inches apart. Your arms should hang loosely at your sides.

2
Inhale as you bend or plié your knees and swing your arms forward and up, over your head. Follow the movement with your eyes, gradually straightening your legs.

3
As you reach the top of the swing, lift your chin slightly, allow your back to arch a bit, and straighten your knees.

Warm up your arms, neck, shoulders, back, and hamstrings with this exercise. You will feel the pull and release of gravity as you swing.

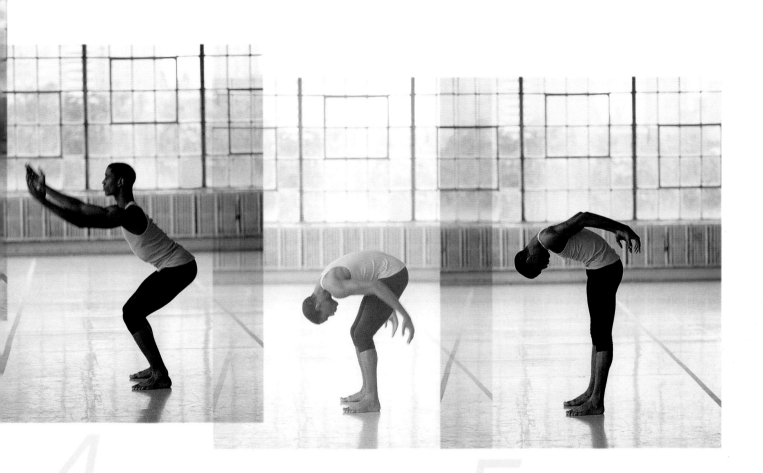

4

In one smooth motion, exhale as you plié and release your arms, swinging them forward and down. Let the momentum of the swing take over, allowing your head, shoulders, and back to follow the downward curve.

5

Straighten your knees as your arms swing behind your legs. Start again at step 2.

Repeat the entire swing-and-release sequence four to six times keeping the movement full. Each swing should happen on a slow count of three; as you warm up, you can increase the speed.

Side-to-Side Lunge

This lunge is a great way to warm up your torso, arms, and ankles.

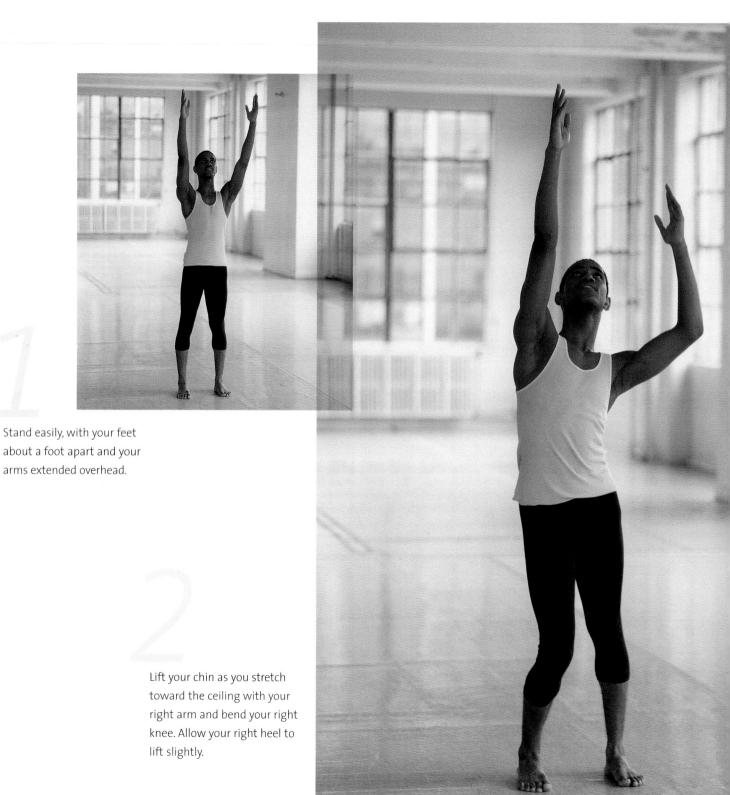

1

Stand easily, with your feet about a foot apart and your arms extended overhead.

2

Lift your chin as you stretch toward the ceiling with your right arm and bend your right knee. Allow your right heel to lift slightly.

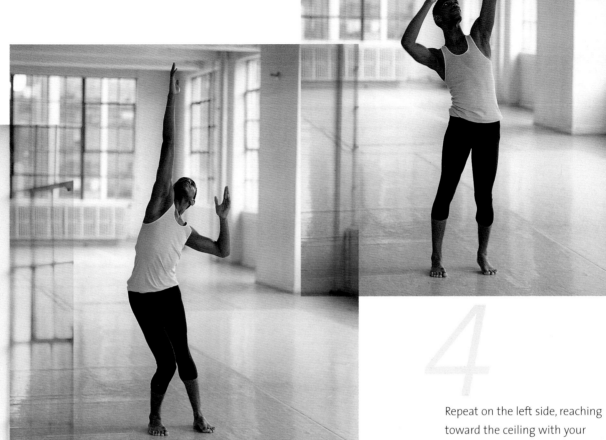

4

Repeat on the left side, reaching toward the ceiling with your left arm, then alternate sides several times, gradually increasing the tempo of your lunges until you establish a comfortable, jazzy rhythm.

3

Keep reaching—imagine your arms are opening up the sky a bit further with every reach. Lower your right heel and allow your left hip to lift slightly. Try to keep your weight distributed evenly over both legs, and keep your knees soft as you knead the floor with your feet.

Deep Plié

The full action of a deep knee bend, or grand plié, engages and warms up the inner thigh muscles, hips, lower back, and abdomen. Move slowly and smoothly and try not to sit at the bottom of the plié.

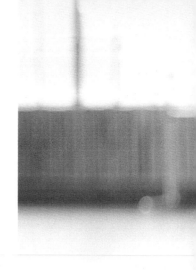

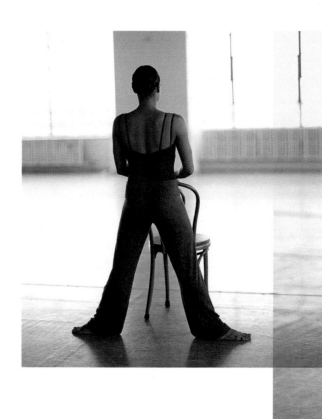

1 Stand in second position, with your legs about shoulder-width apart and your feet open to at least a 45-degree angle.

2 Keep your back upright and your neck long as you slowly bend your knees, opening them over your toes. Try to increase the bending action until your lower legs are perpendicular to the floor. Be careful not to let your body sink into the plié; you want your torso and head to continue reaching up as your knees bend.

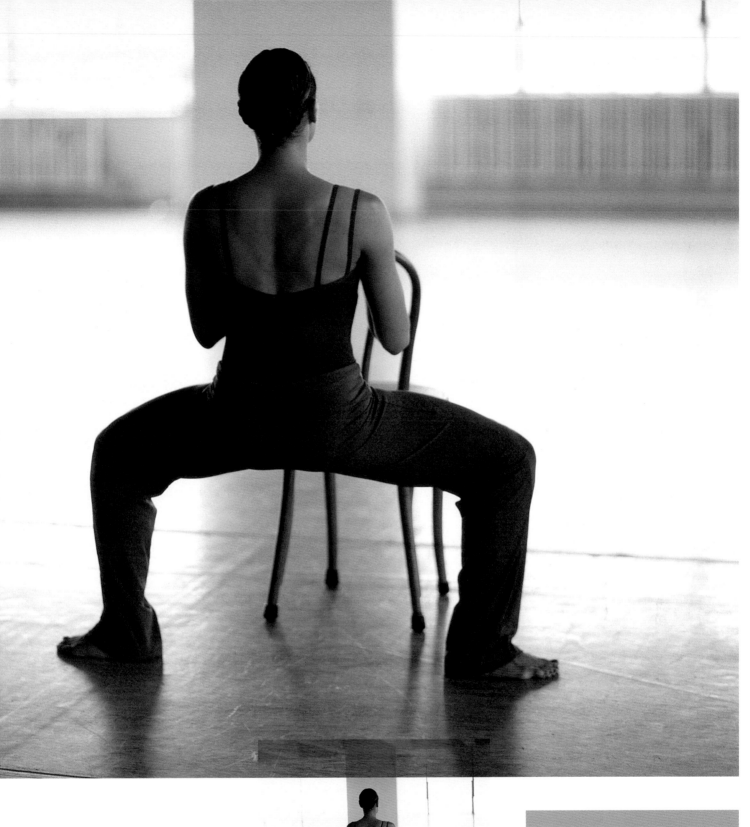

3 Reverse the action, raising your body until your legs are straight.

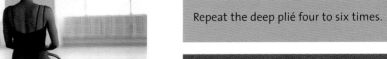

Repeat the deep plié four to six times.

HINT For more stability you may want to hold onto the back of a chair with both hands.

I went to the Jones-Haywood School of Ballet in Washington, D.C., the first black ballet school in the country. Ms. Jones is ninety-something now. To this day, she still inspires and encourages me.

inspirations and influences

My two sisters were heavily involved in dance since they were little. When they changed to a studio where there was a male director and male dancers I saw that it was okay if guys danced, so I joined in.

My fellow dancers inspire me every day, smiling across the way in the wings.

Martha Graham is my greatest inspiration. I love her work, and the fact that she started so late. At the age of twenty-two she took her first dance class.

I saw the Ailey company when I was in high school and said, "That is what I want to do. They really can move, and they are so free."

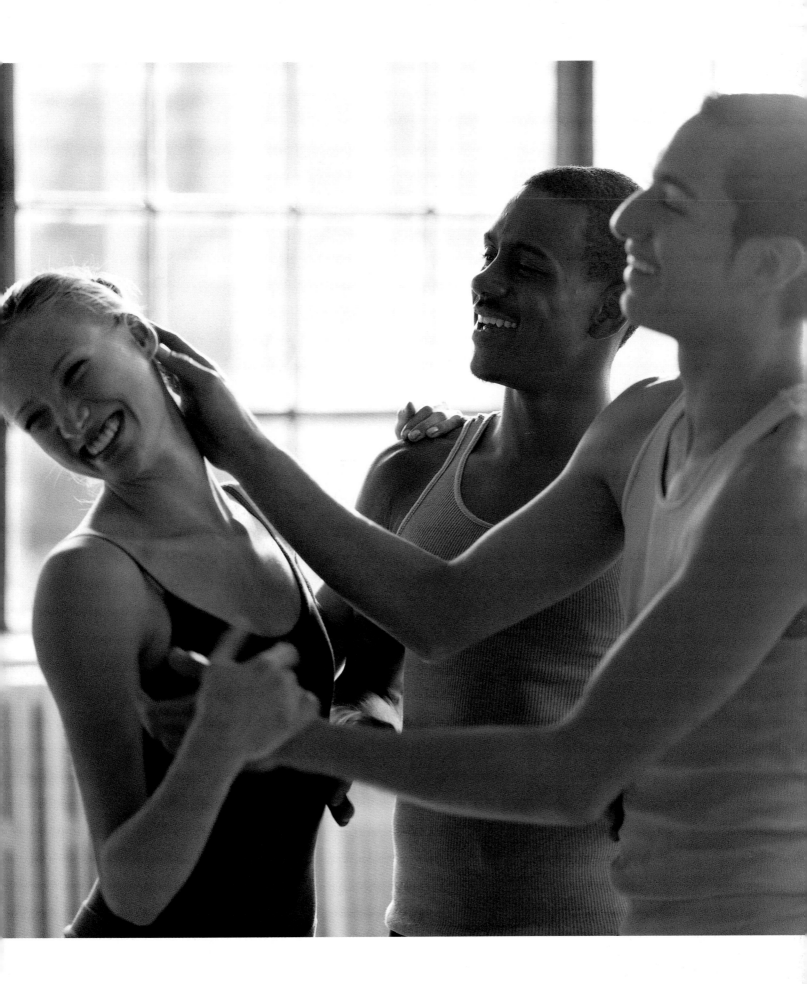

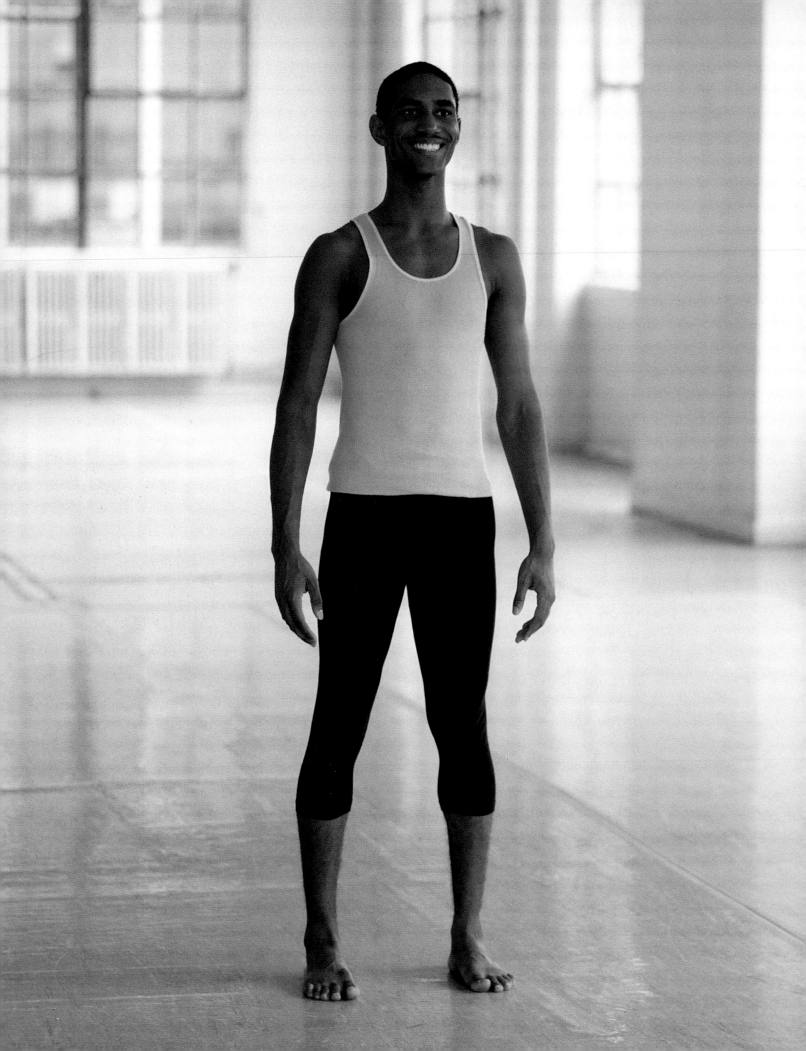

Posture and Alignment

It's easy to spot a dancer walking down the street. There's that unmistakable, strikingly elegant posture. The elongated spine, long neck, and beautifully positioned head radiate physical confidence, tremendous poise, and a sense of purpose. The overall impression is of someone who occupies a slightly exalted position among mortals. Dancers not only look good, their excellent posture makes them healthier. Their bodies are stronger, more comfortable, and more efficient.

Although poor posture is not exactly a federal offense, eventually it will get you into trouble, even if you're not a dancer. A slouching spine and sunken chest telegraph defeat and insecurity; you don't look anywhere near your confident best. Your clothes don't hang properly and you feel lousy. Your back and stomach muscles are weak and your energy sinks into the ground instead of projecting outward. Poor posture means a lack of alignment that inhibits efficient breathing and strains your neck, shoulders, and lower back—and very possibly your knees, ankles, and feet.

While posture habits formed early in life can be especially hard to correct, there are exercises that can help you work effectively with gravity's—as well as daily life's—inexorable pull. But first, take a moment to understand what constitutes correct posture, also known as "neutral alignment," which is the healthiest and most efficient position for your spine. Stand facing a full-length mirror and take a good look.

You're posture-perfect if:
- your head is centered and your ears are level
- your shoulders and hips are level
- your arms hang evenly and easily along your sides
- your knees are level and your kneecaps face forward
- your ankles are straight—no rolling in or out

If viewed in profile, your spine's natural cervical (neck) and lumbar (lower spine) curves should assume a soft S shape. Enlist the help of a photo or supportive friend to see if:
- your head extends up naturally from your spine without jutting forward or tilting backward
- your shoulders are in line with your ears
- your stomach is lifted, not pouching out
- your knees are straight, but not locked
- your lower back forms a gentle forward curve

Here's a good way to gauge whether your cervical and lumbar curves are proper. Stand with the back of your head and buttocks touching a wall. Place your heels two to four inches away from the baseboard. Now, using one hand, feel the distance between your neck and the wall and your lower back and the wall. A couple of inches at your neck and one or two at your lower back are ideal.

Alignment also comes into play while you're seated. To help find the proper alignment of your ears, shoulders, and hips, sit in a straight-back chair and rest your feet on the floor in front of you. Place a small rolled-up towel between the curve of your lower back and the back of the chair—this will support your lower back and ensure the proper position. Strive for the same elongated feeling you had while standing.

Get Your Spine in Line

Floor exercises like this one can help you feel your way to correct alignment. Work slowly and carefully. The differences between the steps are subtle but significant.

2

Breathe deeply. As you exhale, contract your stomach muscles slightly and press your lower back into the floor. Inhale and exhale a few more times, concentrating on the long feeling in your back.

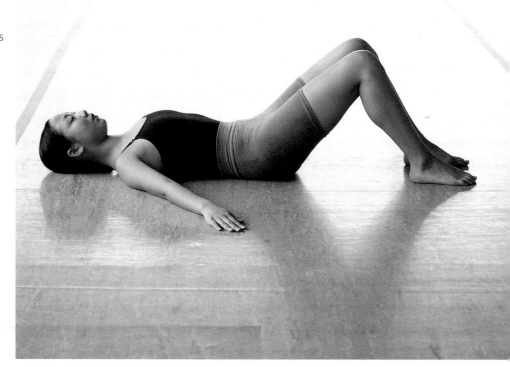

1

Lie on your back with your knees bent in parallel and the soles of your feet flat on the floor near your buttocks. Your arms should be extended along the floor between your hips and waist.

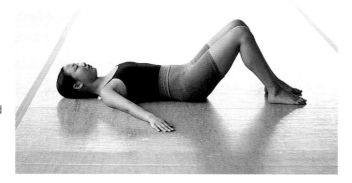

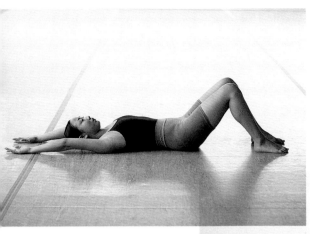

3

Reach overhead with your
arms while keeping your lower
back pressed into the floor.
Release your lower back until
it assumes its natural curve,
slightly away from the floor.

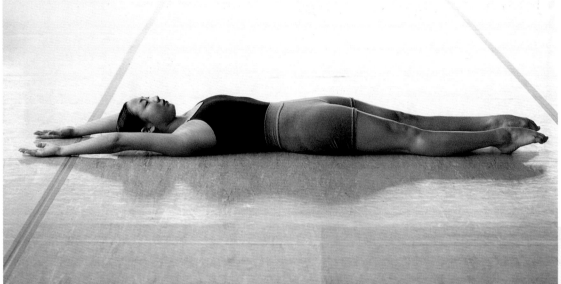

4

Press your back into the floor
again and stretch your legs
along the floor until they are
fully extended.

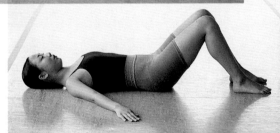

5

Try to keep your back still as
your pull your feet back toward
your buttocks and return your
arms to the starting position.

Repeat the entire sequence three or
four times.

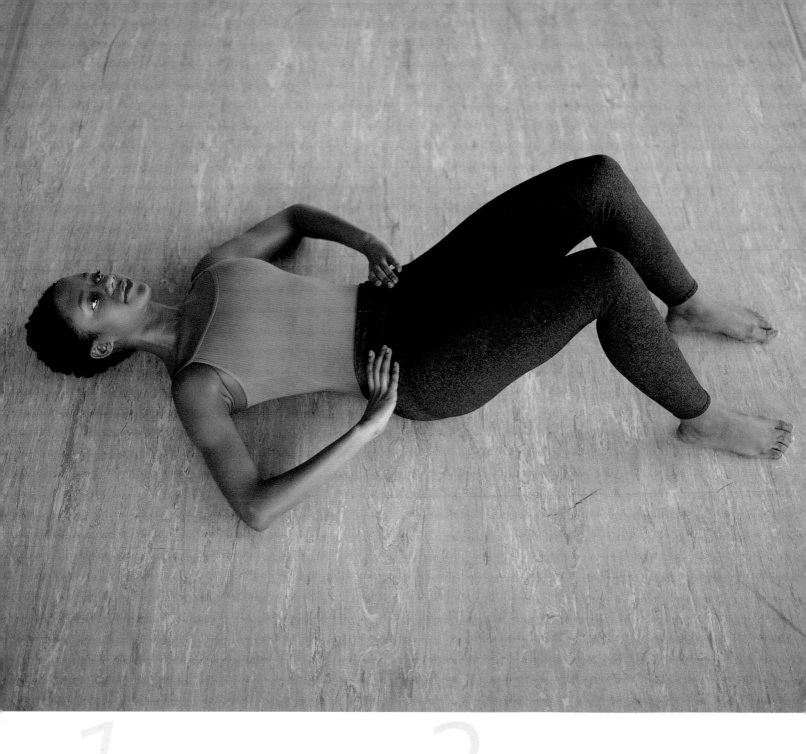

1

Lie on your back with your
knees bent and the soles of
your feet flat on the floor.
Place your hands on top of
your hipbones and rest your
elbows on the floor.

2

Without lifting your elbows off
the floor, push them farther to
the side away from your body
(this is a subtle adjustment).
Hold for a moment, then release
and repeat. You will feel your
upper back open and expand.

Upper Torso Alignment

These deceptively simple upper-body adjustments do wonders for your alignment.

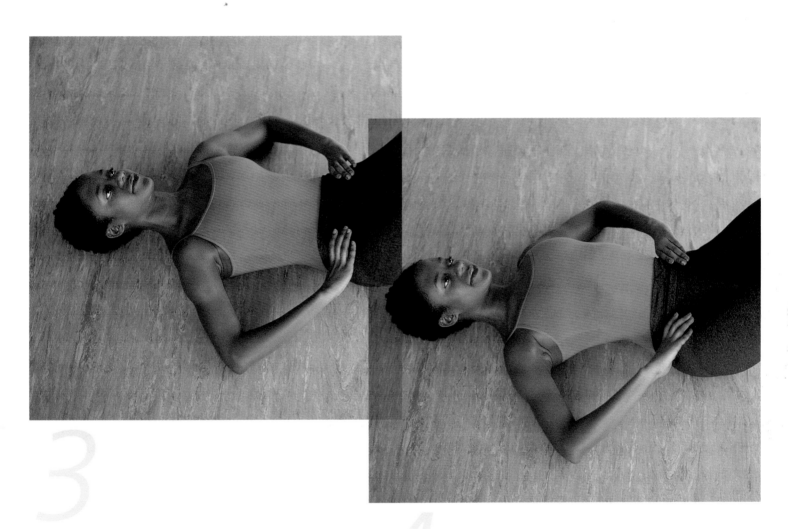

3 Next, keep your elbows on the floor and your back long as you lift your shoulders toward the ceiling. Hold for a moment, then release and repeat. You will feel your neck lengthen.

4 This time lift your rib cage toward the ceiling, allowing your back to arch. Keep your shoulders and hips as still as possible. Hold for a moment, then release and repeat.

Lumbar Sling

A strong stomach is the foundation for a strong back. This gentle and effective exercise works the muscles in your abdomen and waist.

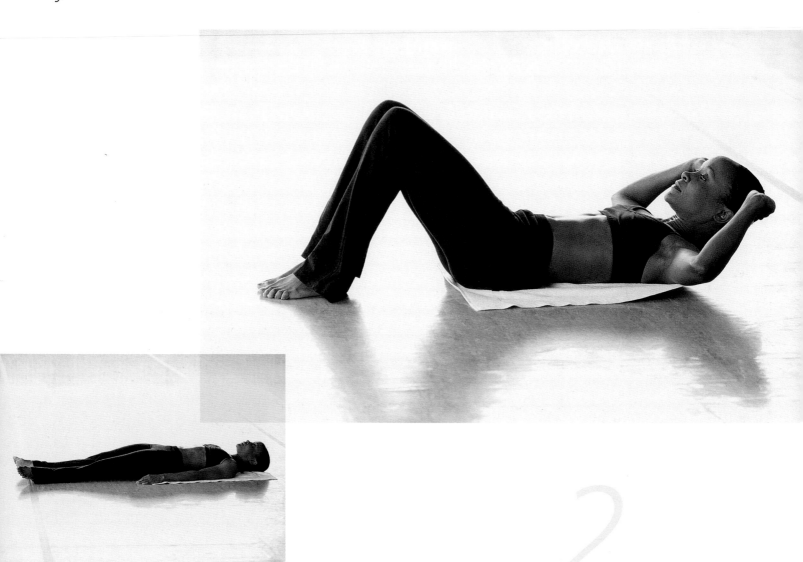

1

Place a bath towel on the floor and lie on top of it, with the crown of your head in line with one short edge.

2

Reach overhead and grab a corner of the towel in each hand. Your knees should be bent and together, the soles of your feet flat on the floor. Inhale, then exhale as you lift your head, neck, and shoulders off the floor. Use the towel as your support.

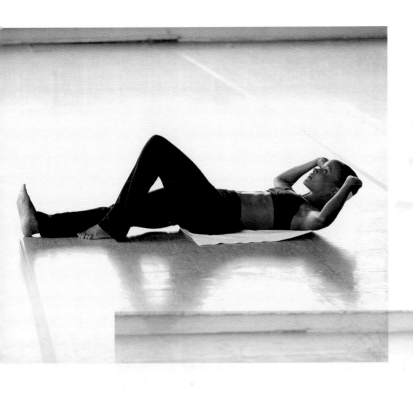

3

Hold this lifted position and inhale as you slide your right heel along the floor until your leg is fully extended.

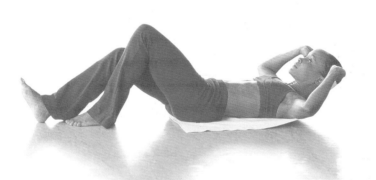

4

Exhale as you pull your heel back toward your buttocks. Concentrate on keeping your abdominal muscles contracted.

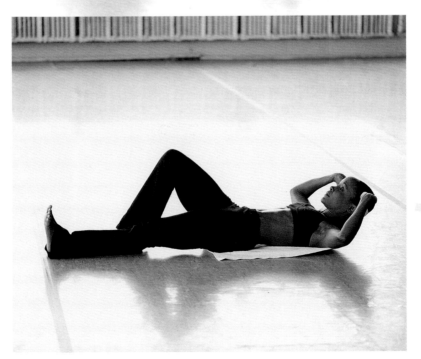

5

Still in a lifted position, repeat with your left leg. Alternate legs 10 to 15 times before lowering your shoulders, neck, and head.

Abdominal Lift

Use your breath and the gentle pulling action
to help activate and lift your abdominals.

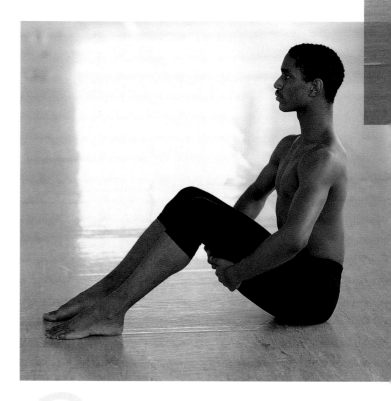

1

Sit on the floor with your knees
bent in parallel and the soles of
your feet flat on the floor. Your
back is slightly rounded and
you are grasping the backs of
your thighs with your hands.

2

Inhale and straighten your
spine, pulling gently against
your thighs.

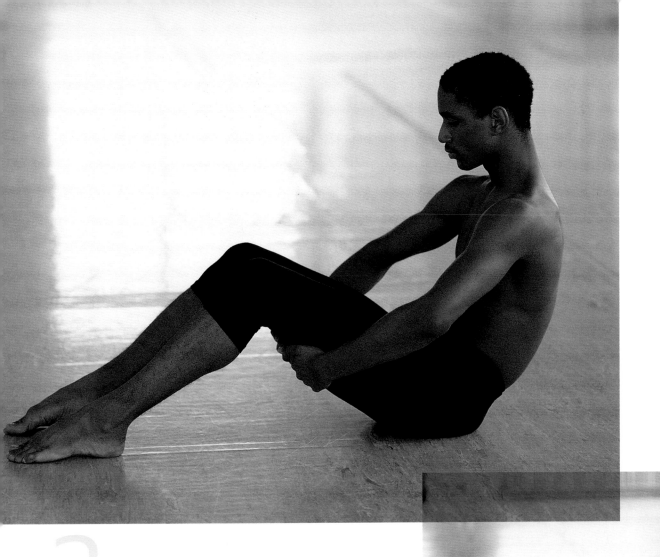

3

Exhale and round your back, pulling your abdomen toward your spine. The action is in your hip joints. Repeat these steps three times.

4

Now add a lift of your chest and head when you straighten your spine. Your sternum reaches toward the ceiling. Repeat these steps, with the lift added, three times.

Basic Spinal Twist

Stretch your spine, pelvis, and hamstrings as you open
up your chest and shoulder girdle with this spinal twist.

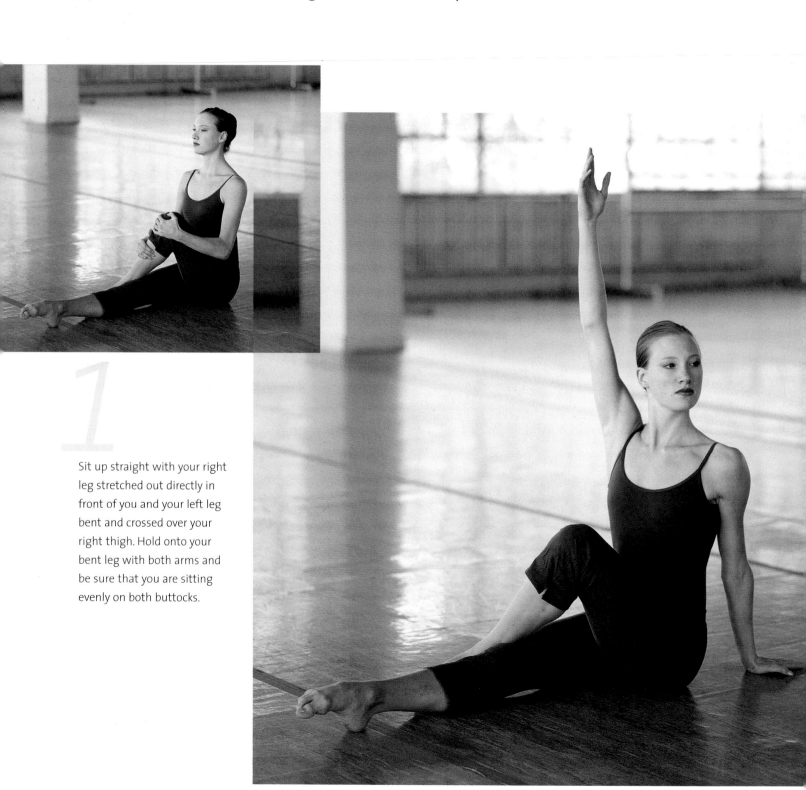

1

Sit up straight with your right
leg stretched out directly in
front of you and your left leg
bent and crossed over your
right thigh. Hold onto your
bent leg with both arms and
be sure that you are sitting
evenly on both buttocks.

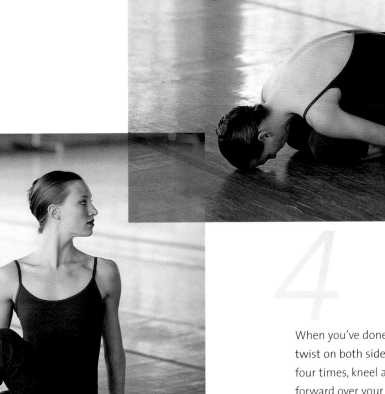

4

When you've done the spinal twist on both sides three to four times, kneel and bend forward over your thighs so your head rests on the floor. In yoga, this is known as Child's Pose. You may want to do this relaxing pose before you begin the exercise as well.

3

Exhale as you lower your right arm in front of your left knee and grasp your left ankle. Turn your head and look over your left shoulder. Hold this twist for a moment. Then untwist, straighten your legs, and repeat with the right leg.

2

Inhale as you raise your right arm straight up and twist your torso to your left. At the same time, place your left hand on the floor behind you for support.

Repeat the exercise on both sides three to four times.

Spinal Curls

This exercise simultaneously strengthens the all-important abdominal muscles and stretches and strengthens your spine.

1

Sit on the floor with the soles of your feet together and your knees open to each side. Your legs and feet should form a triangle. Lightly hold your ankles with your hands and sit up as straight as you can.

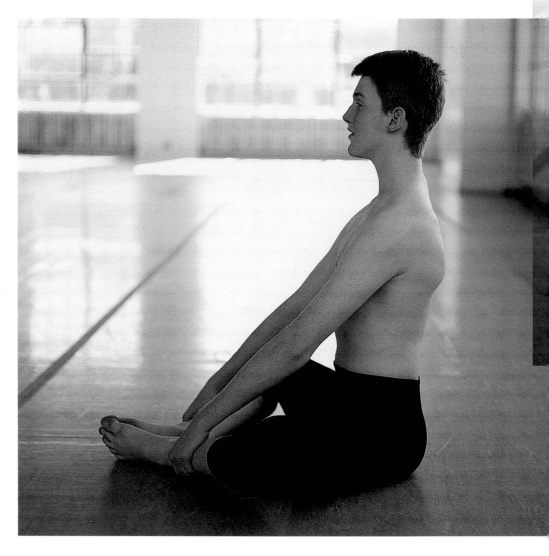

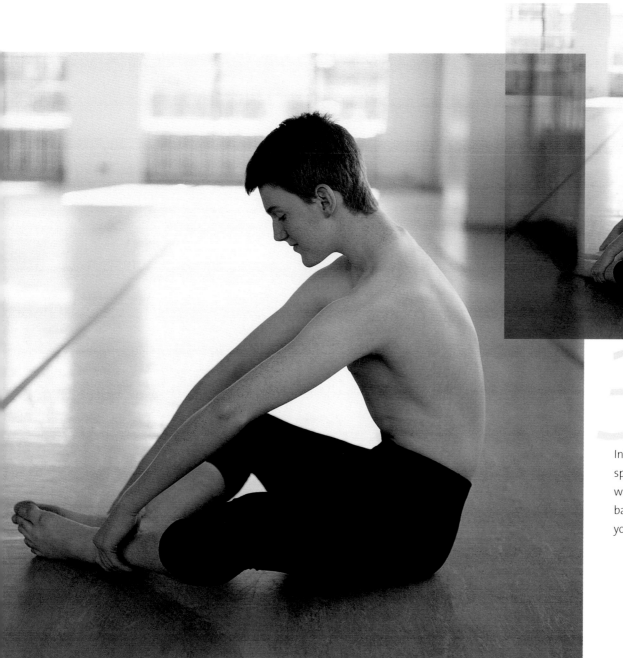

3

Inhale as you straighten your
spine, again beginning at your
waist then lifting your upper
back, neck, and head until
you're sitting tall.

2

Round your spine, starting the
action at your waist, as if someone were pulling your belt from
behind. As you round over,
exhale and curve your upper
back, neck, and head toward
your feet. Keep a light hold on
your ankles.

Repeat this spinal-curl sequence at
least five times. Use your breathing
as impetus for the movement.

Port de Bras

A simple port de bras, a ballet exercise that translates as "carriage of the arms," helps you lengthen and strengthen your upper back and torso.

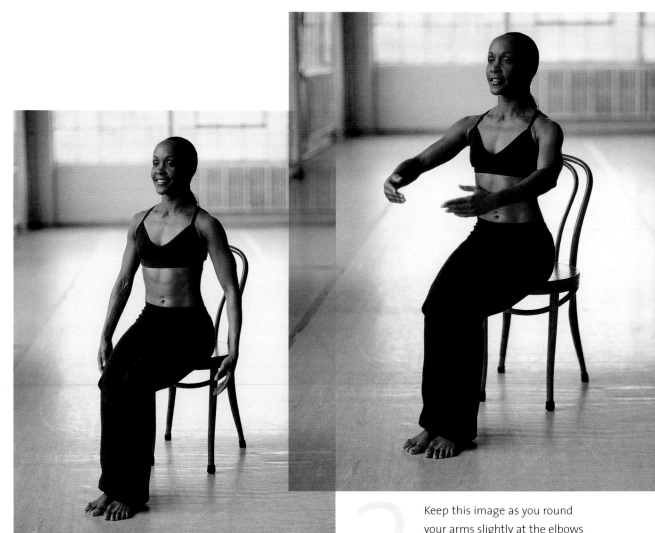

1 Sit up straight with your knees and feet close together and your arms hanging comfortably at your sides. Imagine there's a string coming out of the top of your head, lifting and elongating your neck and spine.

2 Keep this image as you round your arms slightly at the elbows and wrists and slowly move them forward and up until they are in front of your chest. You are holding an imaginary beachball. As you move your arms, try to keep your back long and your stomach lifted. Your shoulders and pelvis should not tip backward.

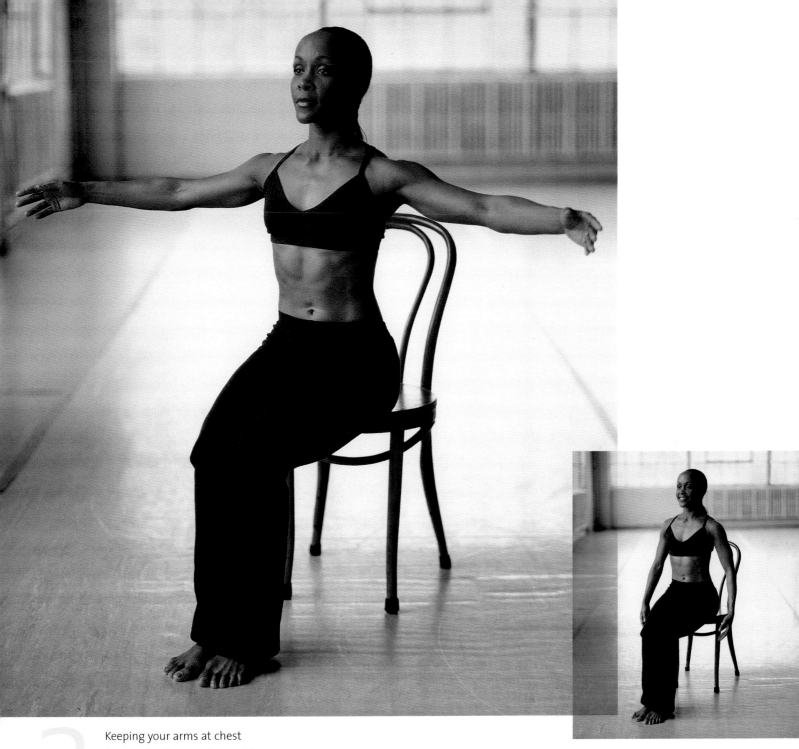

3 Keeping your arms at chest height, slowly open them wide until they're extended to your sides. If you can't see your fingers in your peripheral vision, you've opened too far. Feel the stretch in your torso, but try not to jut your chest out.

4 Lower your arms slowly to your starting position, hanging comfortably at your sides. Repeat three or four times.

HINT Try this exercise in reverse: Lift your arms wide open at chest height, then bring them in front of your chest in a circle and down. Your shoulders should not hike up as you raise your arms.

Hip and Rib Shifts

These subtle isolations of your hips and ribs are a great way to align your spine. Try to keep your upper torso still when you do the hip isolations and your hips still when you isolate your ribs. The thrusting action is sharp and precise.

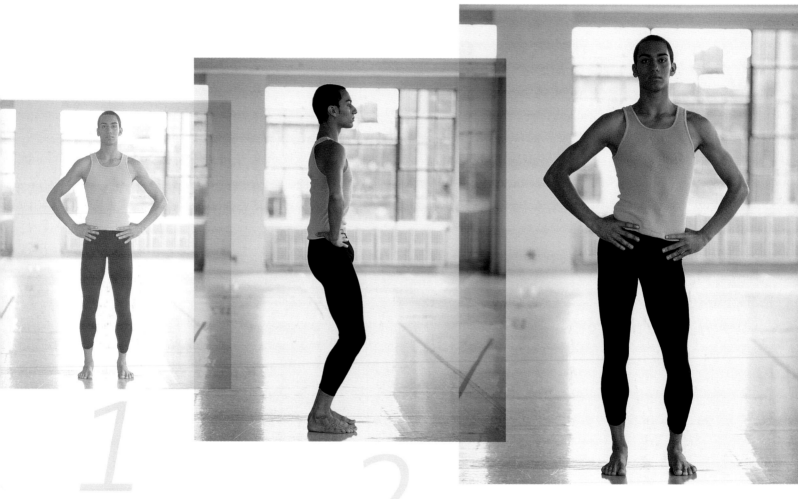

1 Stand with your feet in parallel and your knees slightly bent, in demi plié. Place your hands on your hips. Each photo shows one step of the sequence.

2 Thrust your hips forward, right, back, and left, isolating each movement.

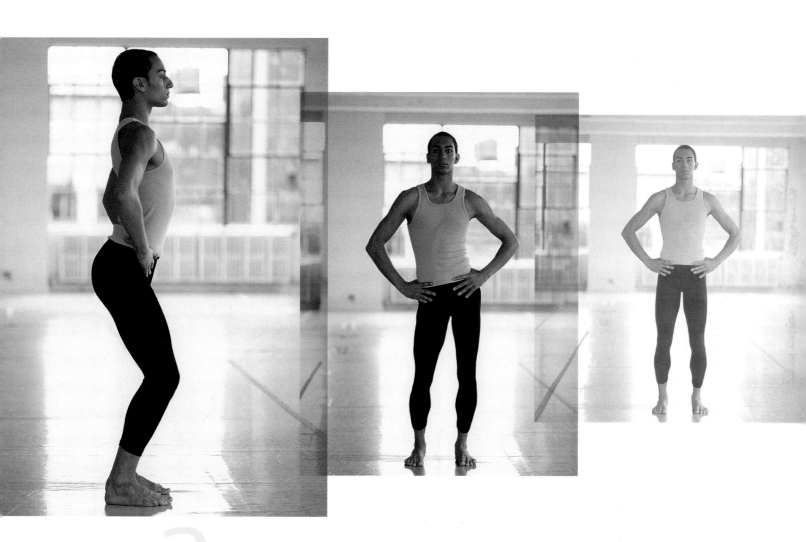

3

When you thrust your hips to the back, be careful that you don't push too far back; you don't want to compress your lower back.

CONTINUED >

Hip and Rib Shifts

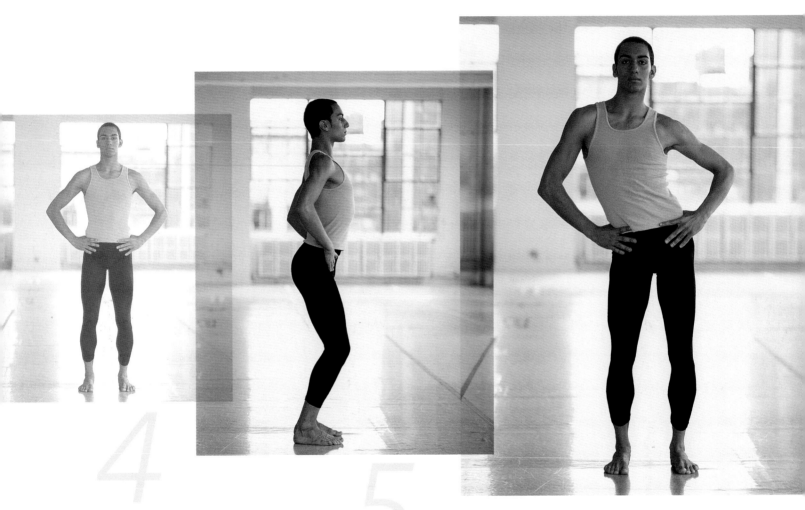

4 Bring your hips back to center, then reverse: forward, left, back, and right. Make sure you don't swivel your knees as you move your hips.

5 Now perform the thrusting isolations with your ribcage, starting to the front, then right, back, and left. Each photo shows one step of the sequence.

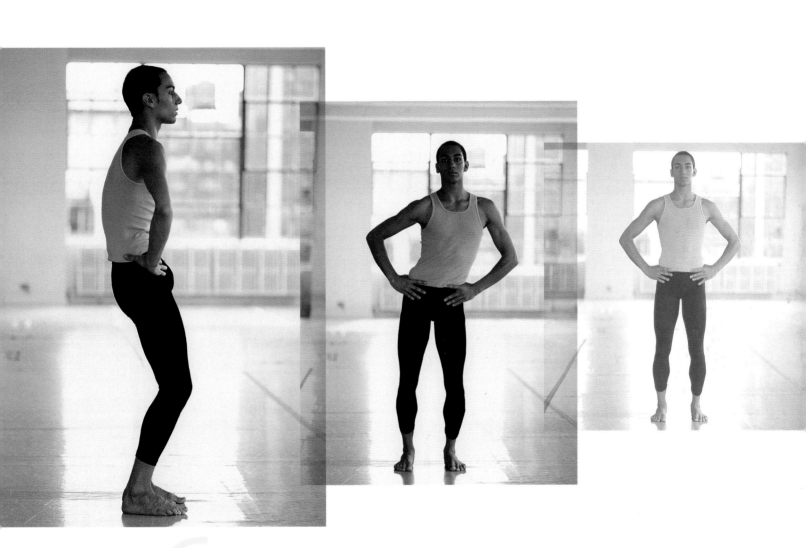

6

Bring your ribs back to center,
then reverse: forward, left, back,
and right. Keep your shoulders
still and your elbows open to
your sides.

Elongate

Here's a great way to do a final check of your alignment.

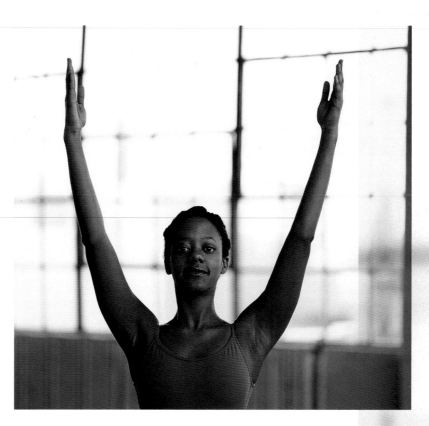

1 Stand with your arms reaching overhead. Your back and neck should be long and your stomach lifted.

2 Lift your shoulders as high as you can—try to touch your ears. Hold this position for a moment as you feel the additional stretch through your rib cage and torso.

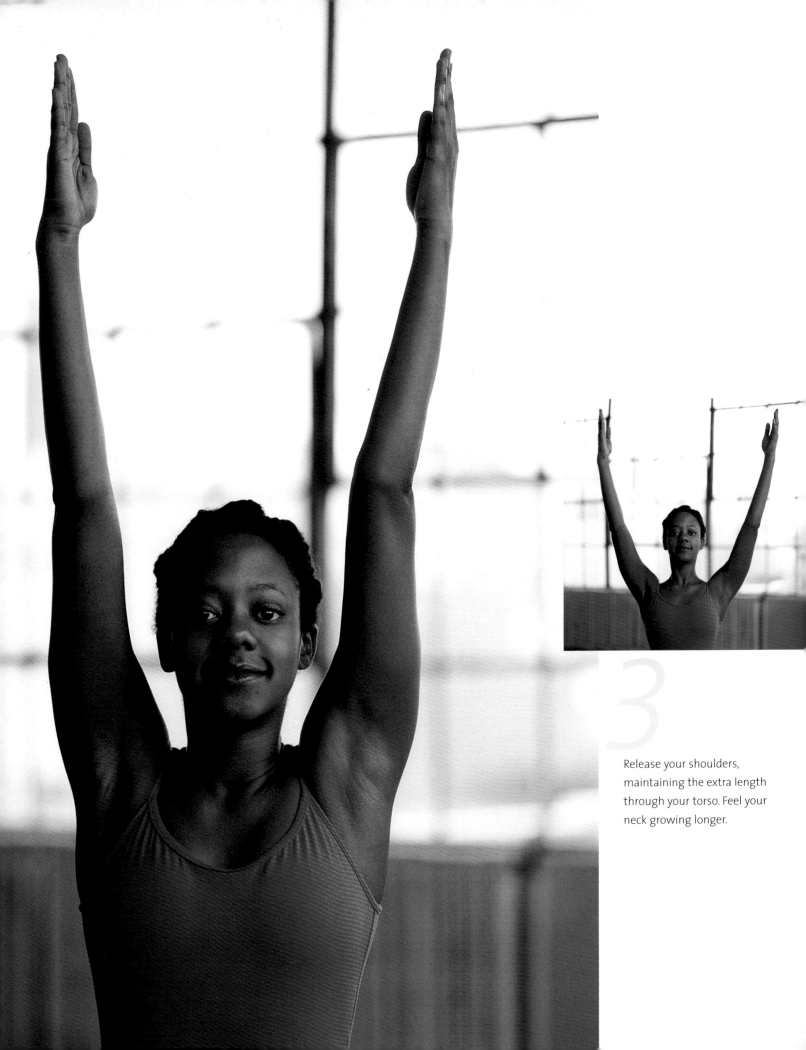

3

Release your shoulders, maintaining the extra length through your torso. Feel your neck growing longer.

I always tell people that you need a passion in life. That's what's important. I'm in love with dance and the art of dance, and I can't deliver anything less than my best because I have respect for myself. *[MR]*

the dancer's life

Renee Robinson and Matthew Rushing

Since I've been in the company so long, when we revisit ballets it's a little more relaxing because I'm familiar with where the movement came from. I've visited a city, been exposed to another culture, or seen a particular exhibit the choreographer mentioned. *[RR]*

I love my work, even on the hard days. I remind myself that even though it's not 9 to 5, dancing is a job. I meet wonderful people. I love the travel. And I remember that there is a goal. *[RR]*

My greatest inspiration is God. *[MR]*

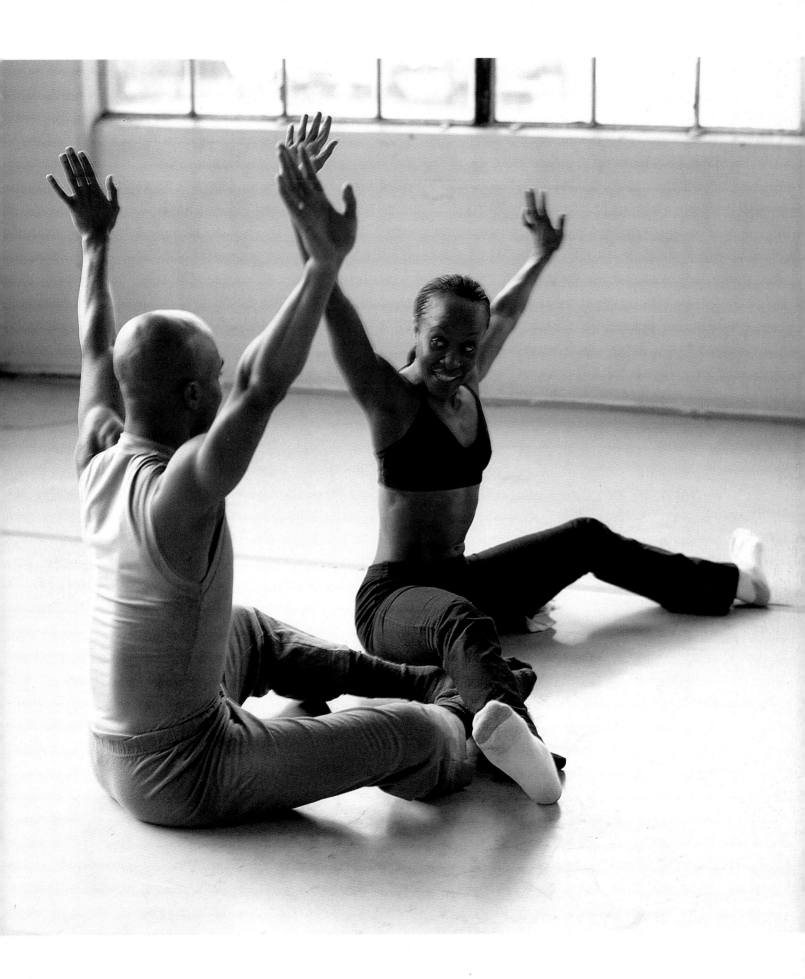

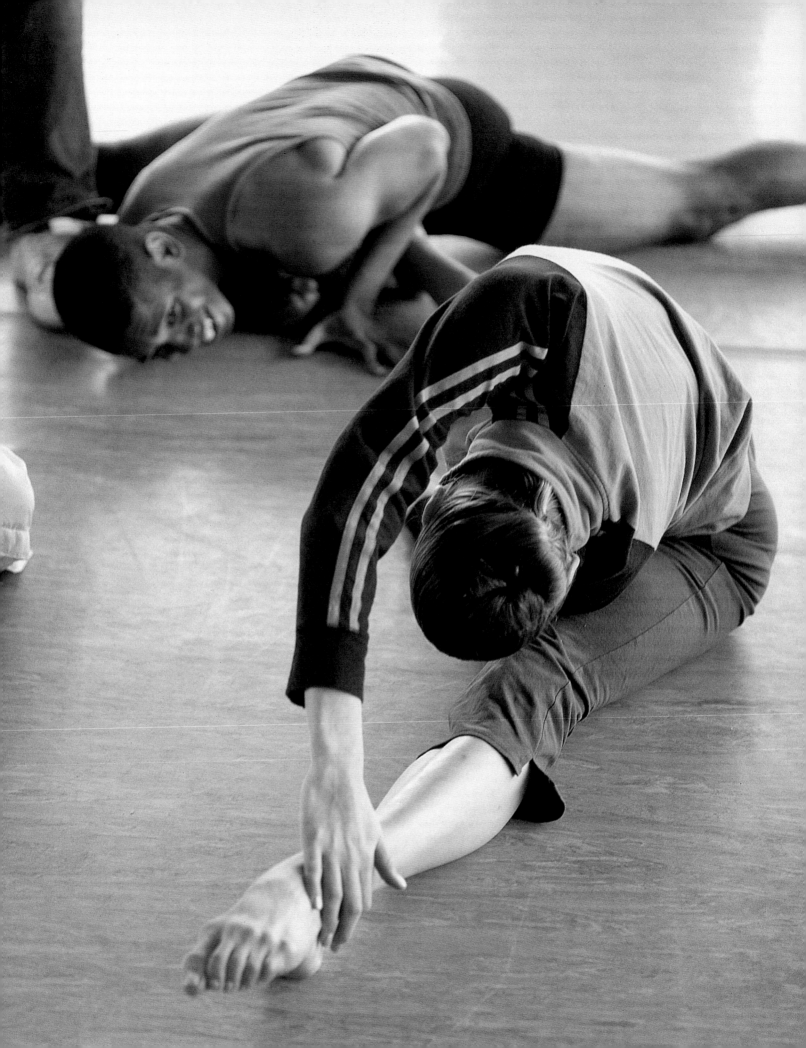

Stretch

When you watch a dancer in action, it may seem like her muscles are made of taffy. There seems to be no limit to how high she can extend her legs or how deeply she can arch her back. The truth is that even dancers who are born with ultraflexible bodies need to devote plenty of quality time to stretching.

Next to warm-up exercises, stretching is perhaps the most important component of your workout routine. Careful, concentrated stretching further prepares your body for movement by increasing your natural range of motion, enabling you to move with greater freedom and flexibility. Stretching also releases muscular tension due to fatigue, overuse, and the inevitable pressures that life throws your way. It is at once relaxing and stimulating to feel your muscles ease into a healthy stretch. Think of stretching as an insurance policy for your muscles. Longer, looser muscles are not only more flexible: because they are more elastic, they are less likely to become injured.

As you stretch, you become aware of which muscles and joints are particularly tight and which are surprisingly supple. Even dancers with muscles like Gumby have a recalcitrant spot or two. Here are several key, dancer-recommended strategies that will help you achieve stretching success.

RELAX. Stretching helps you to relax, but unless you go into it somewhat relaxed, it's a lot harder to derive stretching's many benefits. It's a bit like the story of the chicken and the egg. A thorough warm-up (see page 34) will help you release tension and focus on your stretching routine.

HOLD AND RELEASE. Muscles elongate most effectively when you gently and methodically hold a stretch for 30 seconds or so, then release it, rather than bouncing into the stretch. You'll find that breathing into the stretch—inhaling and exhaling fully—will also help to relax and release your muscles.

STRETCH OFTEN. Stretching is most beneficial when you do it frequently and consistently. You should stretch after your warm-up, in between strengthening exercises, and as part of your post workout cool-down. A slightly fatigued muscle relaxes and lengthens more easily.

BE PATIENT. It's great to try to kick your leg up to your ear, but increasing your range of motion takes time. Gradual and methodical stretching, going a little farther each day, is what yields results.

BE GENTLE. Forcing your muscles into a stretch is not only risky—you could end up with a whopper of an injury—it's painful. Remember, your muscles are not rubber bands: they are living fibers with memories and limits. Stretch slowly and with control. If a stretch starts to hurt, ease up. Tomorrow is another day.

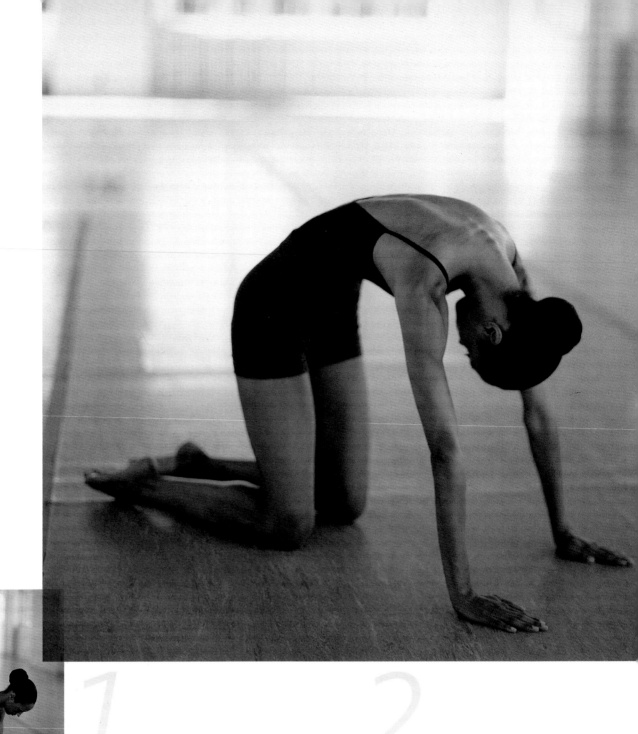

1

Start on your hands and knees.
Your back and neck should be
long; your hands should be
directly under your shoulders
and your knees directly under
your hips.

2

Inhale, then exhale as you
round your back and pull your
stomach toward your spine.
Allow your neck and head to
complete the curve.

Cat

Stretch your spine like a cat. You may find this exercise more comfortable if you place a folded towel or small pillow under your knees.

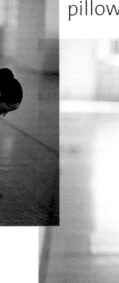

3

Inhale as you release the curve and move through your starting position.

4

Keep moving as you exhale, slowly arching your back and lifting your chin. Be sure that you don't drop into the arch: the movement throughout the exercise should be continuous and fluid.

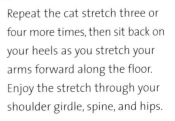

5

Repeat the cat stretch three or four more times, then sit back on your heels as you stretch your arms forward along the floor. Enjoy the stretch through your shoulder girdle, spine, and hips.

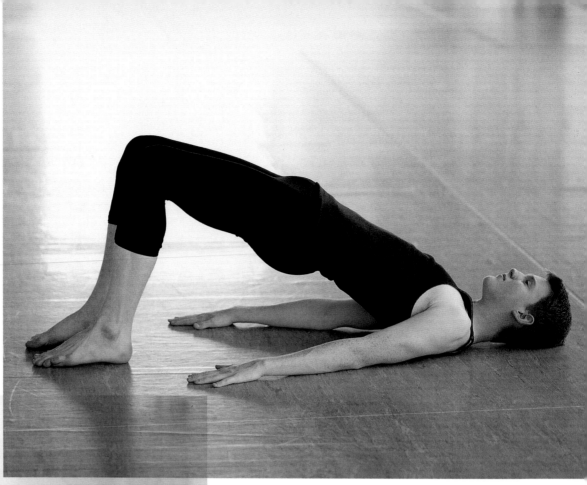

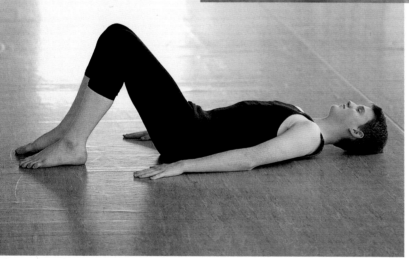

2

Gently lift your pelvis, pressing it toward the ceiling. Keeping your upper back and shoulders on the floor, inhale and exhale.

1

Lie on your back with your knees bent and the soles of your feet flat on the floor. Your arms should be stretched along your sides with your palms on the floor.

Hip Lift

This exercise stretches your hips, lower back, and the quadriceps (the four interdependent muscles that run along the front of each thigh).

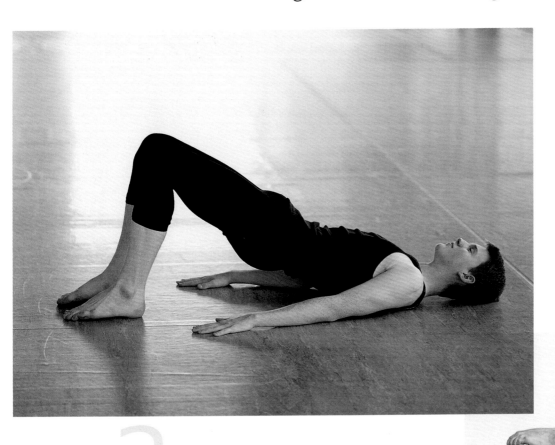

3

Lower your pelvis, slowly rolling down through your spine until you are in your starting position.

4

Repeat the hip lift three times, then hug both knees to your chest until your hips are lifted slightly off the floor. Feel the stretch through your buttocks.

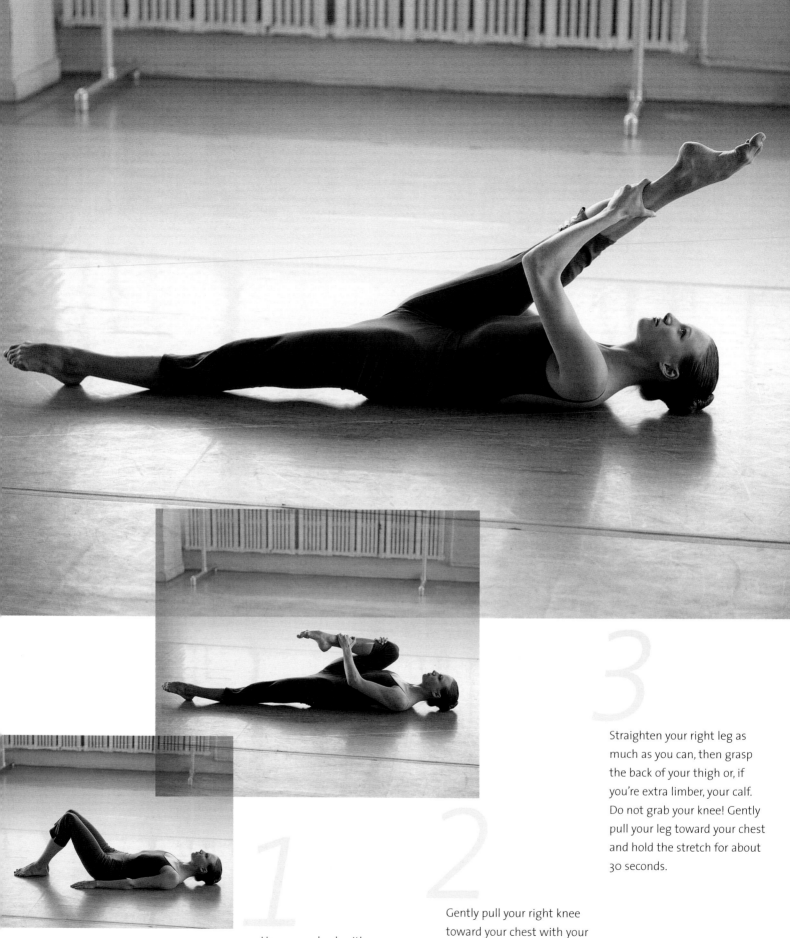

3

Straighten your right leg as much as you can, then grasp the back of your thigh or, if you're extra limber, your calf. Do not grab your knee! Gently pull your leg toward your chest and hold the stretch for about 30 seconds.

2

Gently pull your right knee toward your chest with your hands, and extend your left leg along the floor.

1

Lie on your back with your knees bent and the soles of your feet flat on the floor.

Hamstring Stretch

Hamstrings are often very tight; they require thorough stretching.

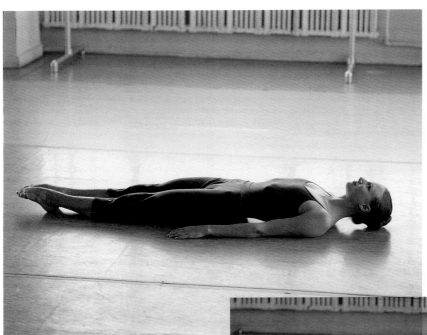

4

Carefully lower your leg to the floor, counterbalancing it with a strong, scooped-out abdomen (see page 115).

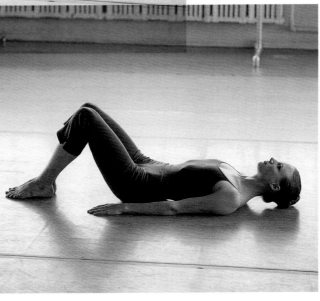

5

Bring your leg back to your starting position and repeat the hamstring stretch on your left side.

"Number 4" Stretch

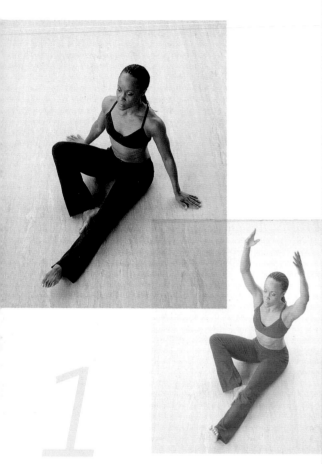

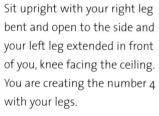

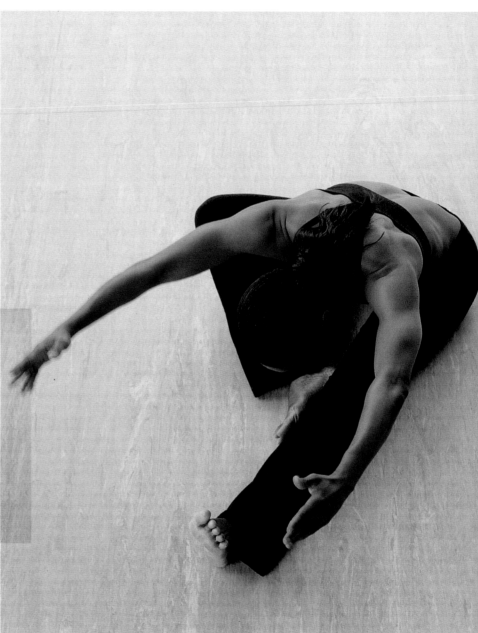

1 Sit upright with your right leg bent and open to the side and your left leg extended in front of you, knee facing the ceiling. You are creating the number 4 with your legs.

2 Inhale as you flex your left foot and lift your arms overhead, reaching up and out.

3 Exhale and slowly round your back over your left leg. Hold this position for a moment, then roll up slowly through your spine. You should be in the starting position again.

This exercise stretches your back, hips, legs, ankles, and feet.

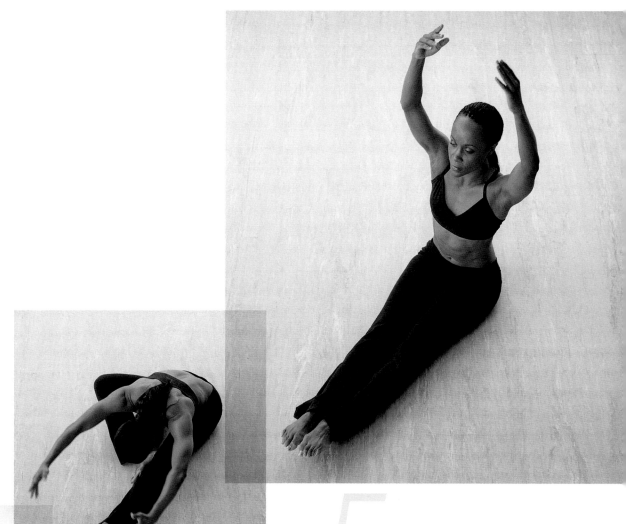

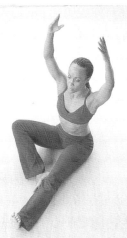

4

Repeat this entire sequence, this time with your left foot pointed.

5

Switch sides and repeat, then, if you're up for an extra challenge, repeat the entire sequence with both legs extended forward.

Hanging Stretch

Let the weight of your torso and head help you stretch. Breathe deeply and hold each position for eight slow counts.

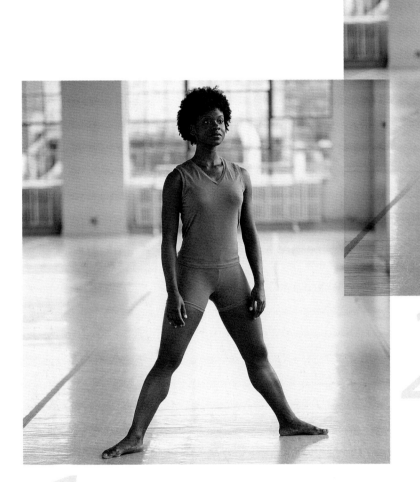

1

Stand with your legs in second position and your arms hanging comfortably at your sides.

2

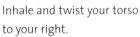

Inhale and twist your torso to your right.

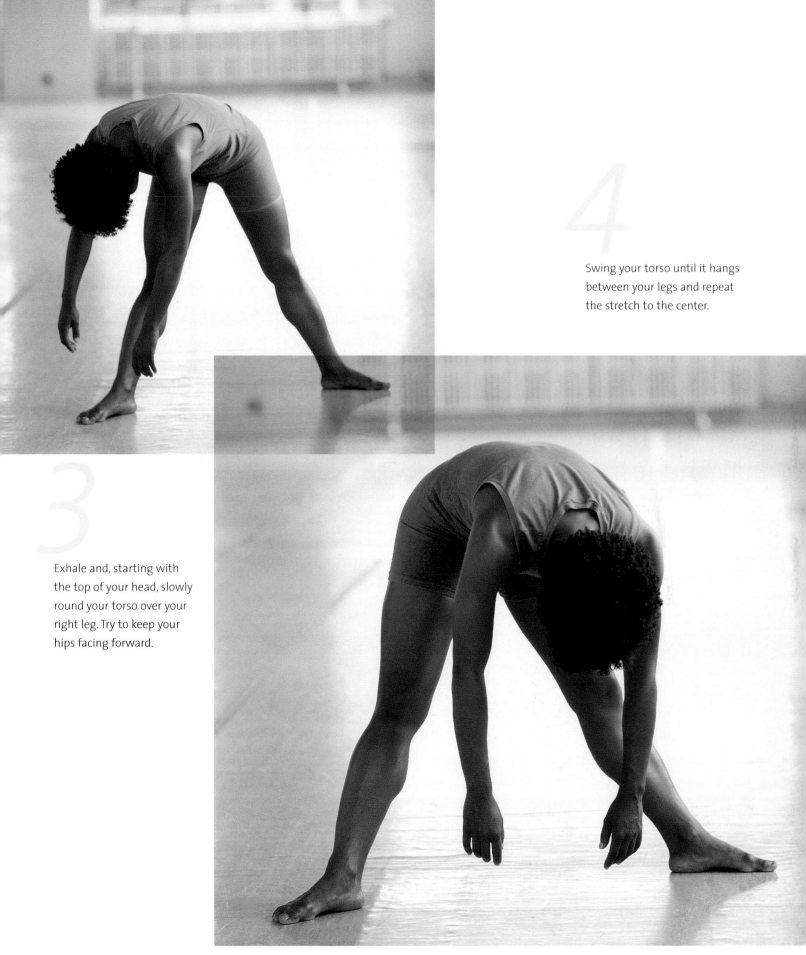

4

Swing your torso until it hangs between your legs and repeat the stretch to the center.

3

Exhale and, starting with the top of your head, slowly round your torso over your right leg. Try to keep your hips facing forward.

CONTINUED >

Hanging Stretch

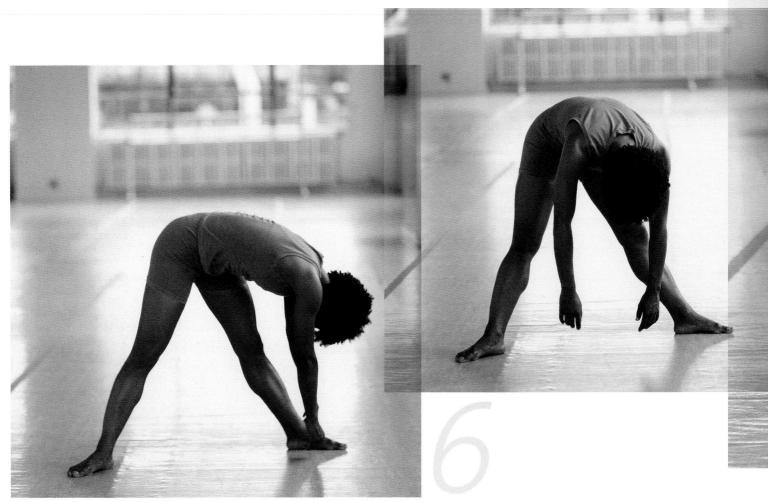

5 Swing your torso over your left leg and repeat the stretch.

6 Swing it back to the center and stretch again.

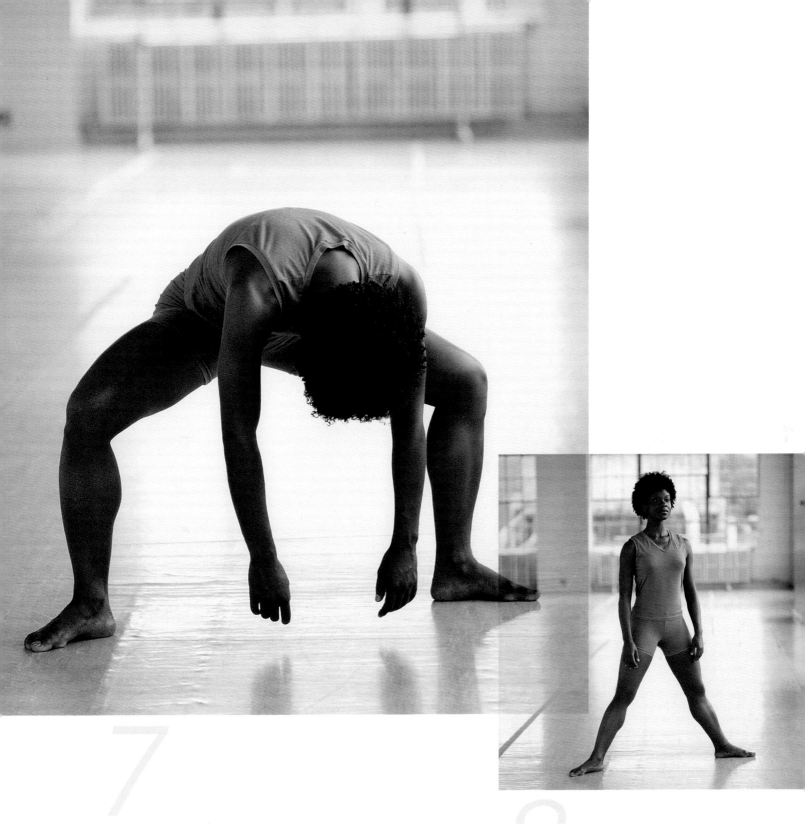

7

With your torso still rounded over, plié, bending your knees four counts down, and four counts up. Be careful to keep your knees over your feet. Feel the stretch through your inner thighs. Repeat two more times.

8

When you've finished, bend your knees slightly as you roll up slowly through your spine, vertebra by vertebra, until you're standing.

Lunging Stretch

Stretch your quadriceps and hamstrings with these lunges.

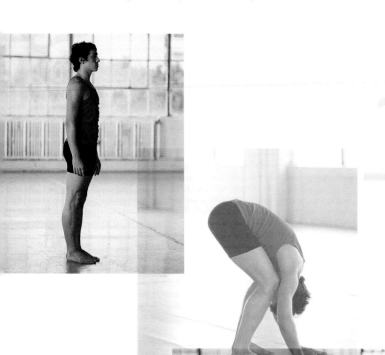

1 Starting with your feet parallel and together, plié, bending your knees until you can place both hands on the floor in front of your feet. Allow your torso to curl forward and your heels to lift off the floor as you bend.

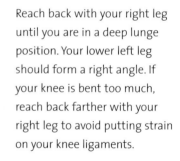

2 Reach back with your right leg until you are in a deep lunge position. Your lower left leg should form a right angle. If your knee is bent too much, reach back farther with your right leg to avoid putting strain on your knee ligaments.

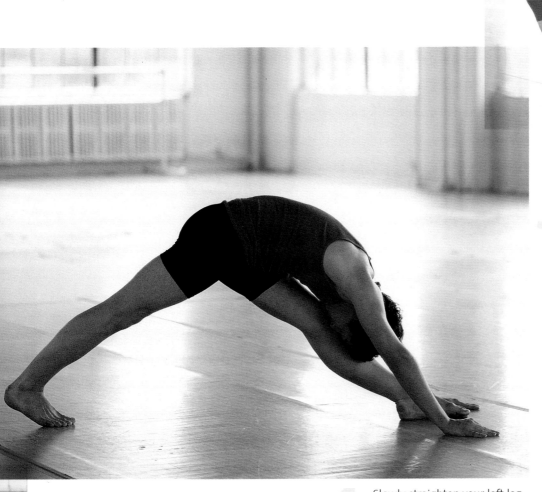

5 Bring your right leg forward to meet your left and roll up to the starting position. Repeat the lunge sequence, this time with your left leg reaching back.

4 Slowly straighten your left leg as much as possible and curve your torso over your left leg. You can place your fingertips on the floor for support. If you can't touch the floor, bend your left knee a bit more until you can. Hold for about one minute. Remember to breathe.

HINT When you've finished your lunge, keep your knees slightly bent as you roll up slowly through your spine.

3 Place your hands on either side of your left leg and gently press your pelvis toward the floor. Try to keep your neck long as you lift your gaze forward. Hold the stretch for 30 seconds to one minute.

Calf Stretch

Your calves require a gentle but firm stretch.

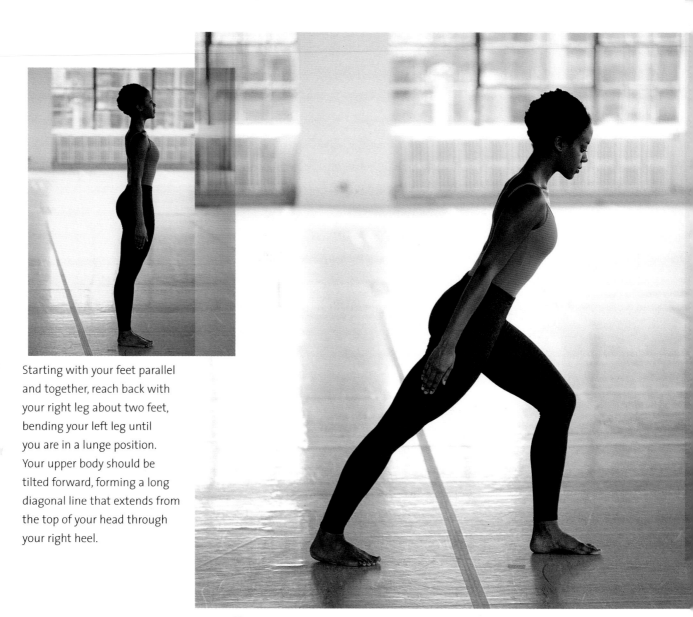

1 Starting with your feet parallel and together, reach back with your right leg about two feet, bending your left leg until you are in a lunge position. Your upper body should be tilted forward, forming a long diagonal line that extends from the top of your head through your right heel.

2 Keep your body weight over your left leg and press your right heel toward the floor, taking care that your right foot doesn't turn out or in. Hold this position for about 30 seconds. You will feel a powerful stretch through your calf muscle.

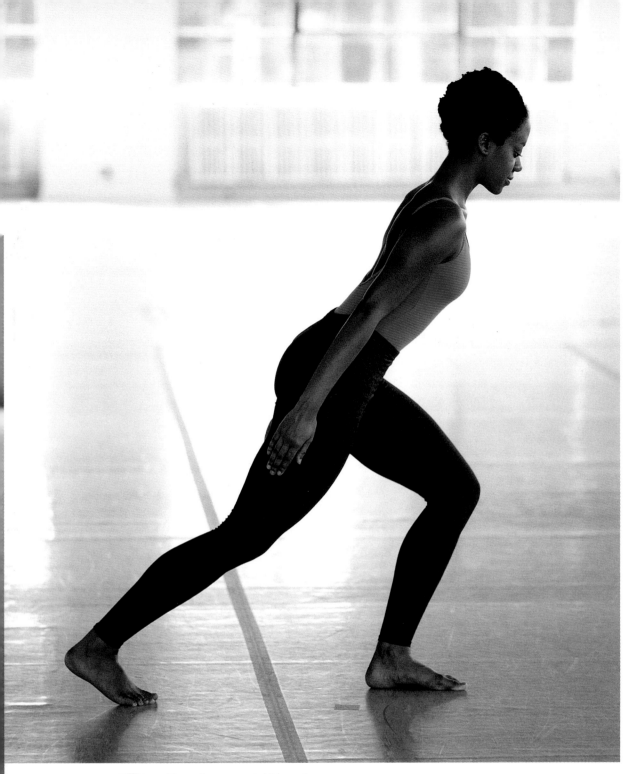

3 Now allow your right knee to bend. If your heel lifts off the floor slightly, that's fine. Hold the stretch and feel it move through your calves and into your shins.

Repeat the calf-stretch sequence on your left side.

HINT If you have trouble balancing, you can place your hands against a wall for support. Be sure to keep your shoulders level.

Torso Tilt

Stretch your torso, shoulder girdle, and arms with this exercise. Use the strength in your abdominals to maintain the alignment through your torso.

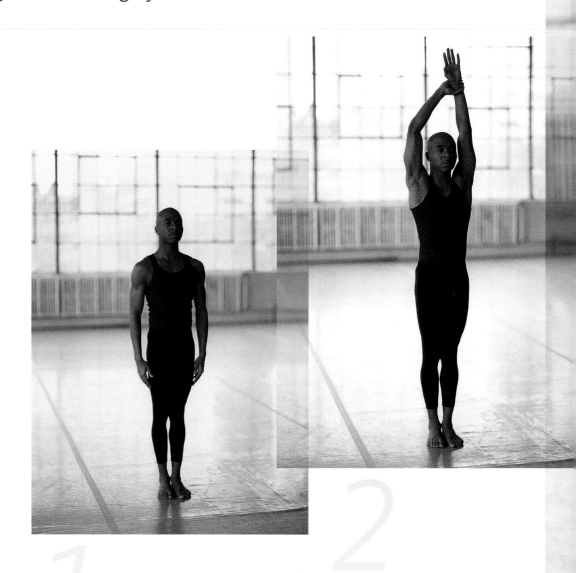

1

Stand with your feet parallel and together and raise your arms over your head. Your shoulders should be down and relaxed and your neck and back long.

2

Grasp your left hand with your right, reaching higher as you tilt your torso to your right. Keep your pelvis facing forward and try not to sink into your left hip or twist your torso as you tilt. Watch that you don't hike up your shoulders.

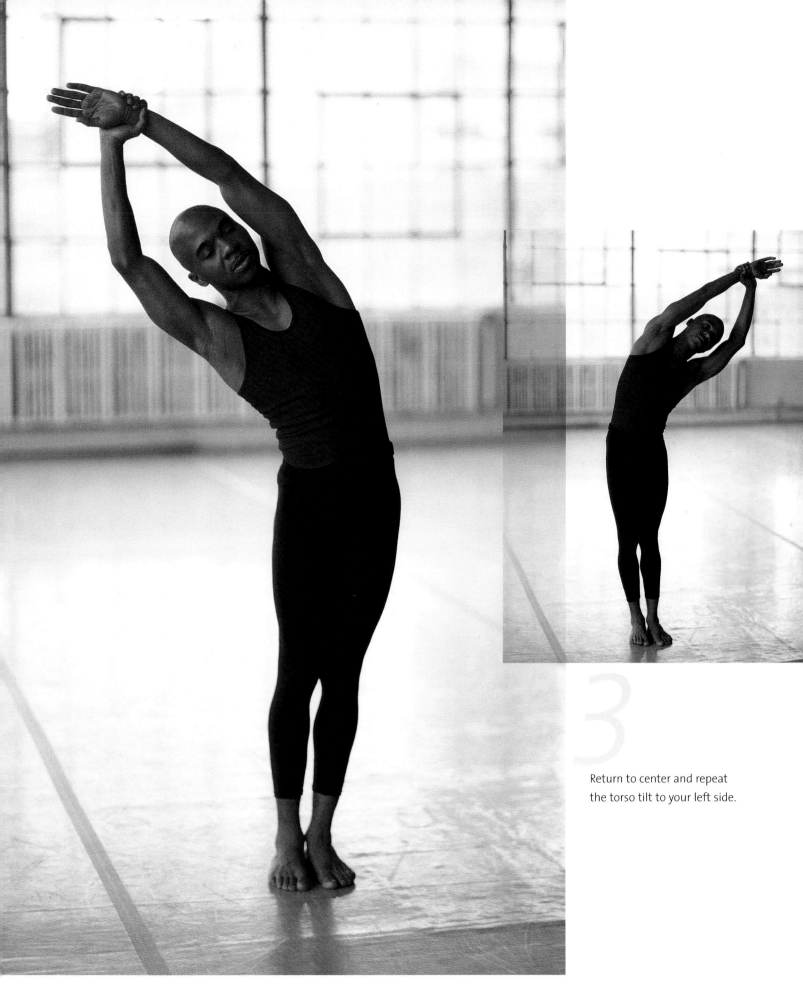

3

Return to center and repeat
the torso tilt to your left side.

Handiwork

Stretch your lower arms, hands, and fingers with these exercises, which can be done seated or standing. Do each movement in three slow, steady counts.

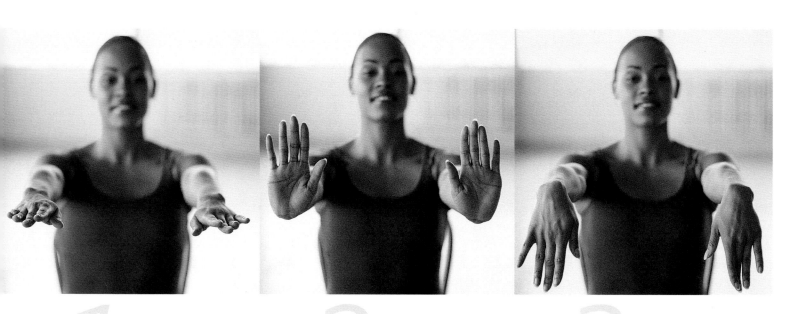

1

Raise your arms in front of you to chest height. Your palms should face the floor and your fingers should be extended, creating a long line from your shoulders through your finger-tips. Keep your shoulders down and relaxed and your neck and back long.

2

Lift your fingers toward the ceiling. Keep your fingers together, and your arms and torso as still as possible.

3

Press your fingers downward, passing through your starting position until your fingertips are pointed toward the floor.

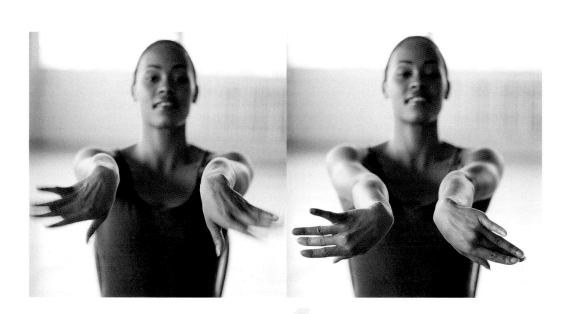

4

Next circle your fingers, four times outward and four times inward. Allow your fingers to splay so you can get the maximum stretch in every direction.

CONTINUED >

Handiwork

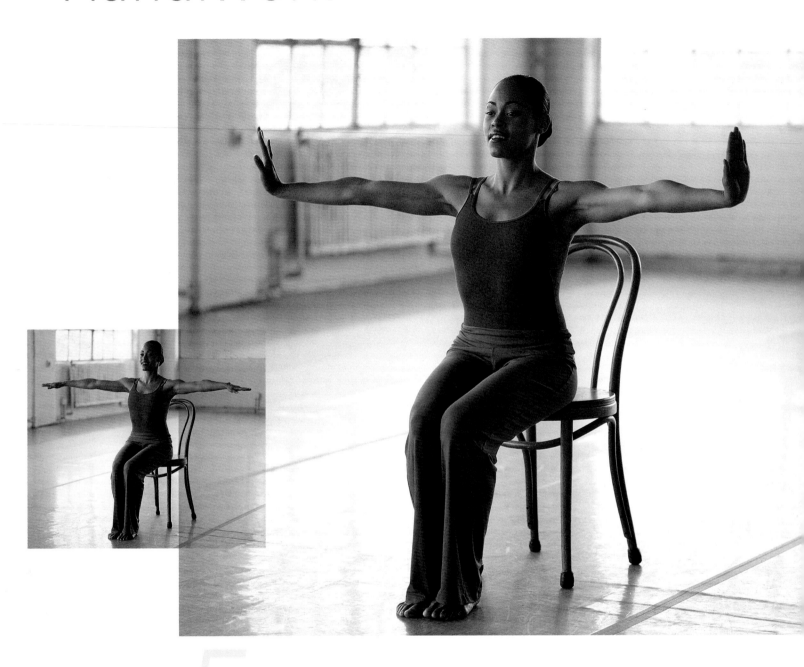

5

Repeat two times, then try the
same exercise with your arms
extended to your sides.

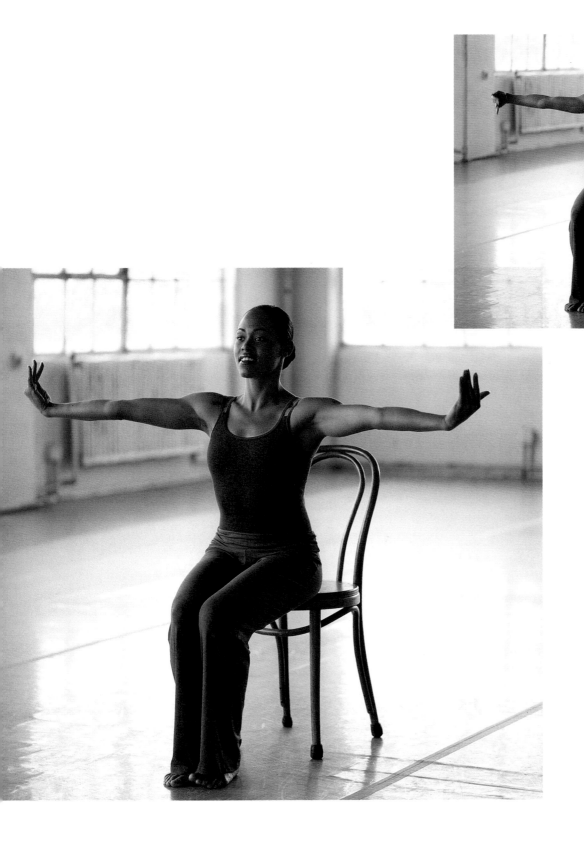

I love to move, so it's easy for me to get out of bed and go to class every day. It's a wonderful job. We are getting paid to make crazy shapes.

energizers

Stay connected to family and friends. Read the newspaper.

Music in the morning gets me going—some gospel or hip-hop to get the blood moving, the energy flowing.

Treat yourself to chocolate every now and again.

It's a mental thing—pacing yourself, eating small meals throughout the day. I've learned to have raisins, fruit, and nuts for snacks.

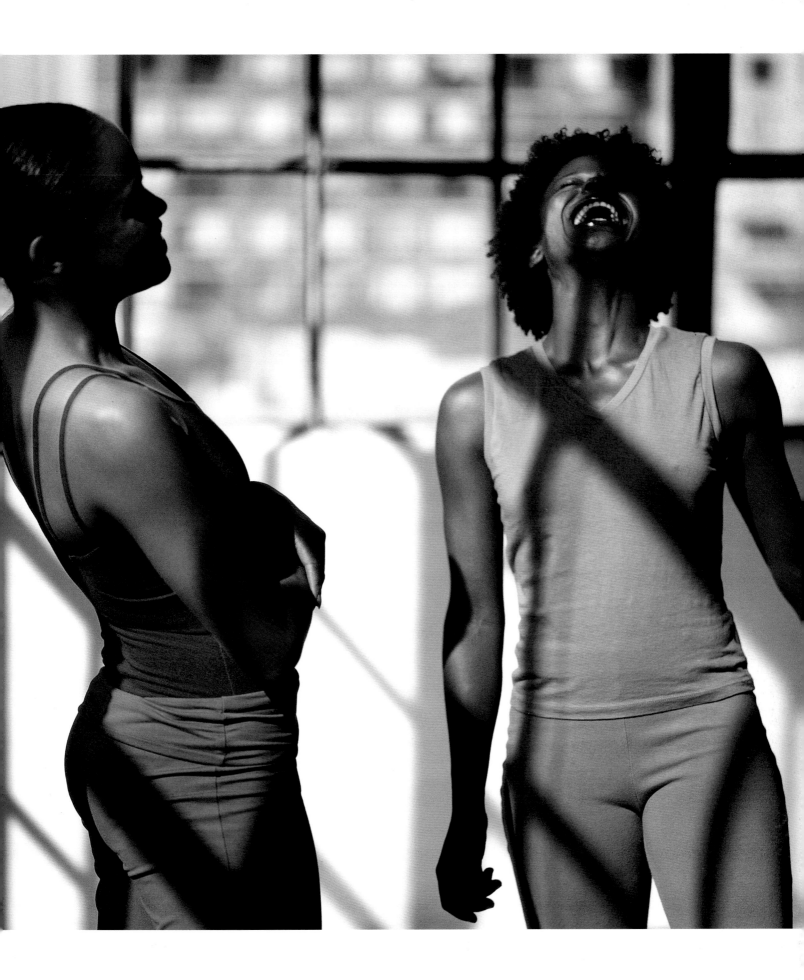

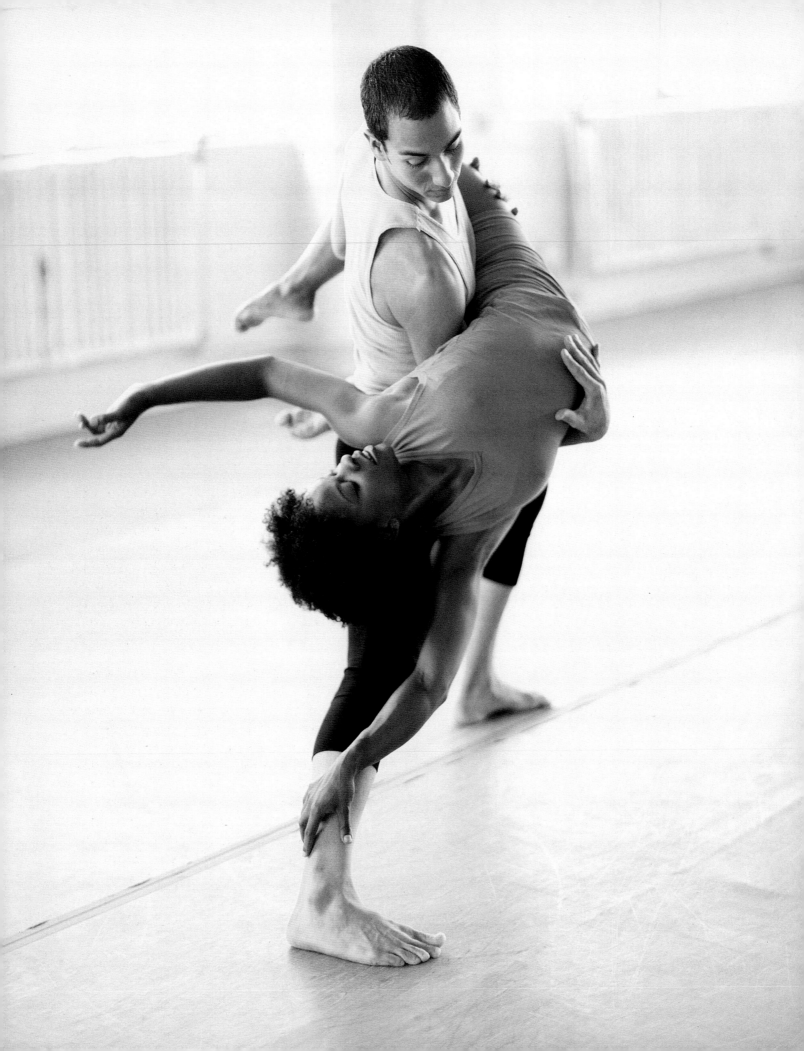

Strength

Strength is more than the ability to hoist heavy weights; it is the sum of your energy. A strong body defines your presence. A body without strength can't stand up on its own, much less move. Strength enables you. It is the muscular wherewithal to get the job done. And, along with stretching, it is a barrier to exhaustion and injury.

Just as with stretching, the process of getting stronger—putting your muscles through their various paces—requires mental as well as physical focus. Actively engaging your attention and tuning in to how your own body responds to a particular exercise will yield far greater results than a more haphazard approach.

For a dancer, strength is the key to endurance, power, and control. A stratospheric leap requires tremendous muscular oomph, as does the ability to mesmerize with a gyroscopic balance. Dancers in general aren't particularly interested in developing tremendously bulky muscles. In fact, most prefer the more elegant, streamlined look of muscles that have gained their strength through exercise that uses the weight and force of their own bodies working against the push and pull of gravity.

Strengthening—the contracting and shortening of muscles—is the codependent partner of stretching. Your muscles are healthiest when you balance one with the other. Some of this strategic pairing happens during the course of a single movement. When you lift your leg to the front, for example, you're strengthening your quads and stretching your hamstrings: One muscle group relaxes to enable the opposite set to contract. Incorporate frequent, careful stretches into your strengthening routine, and you'll not only gain flexibility, you'll stave off injury and increase your ability to respond quickly and efficiently to the demands of a wide variety of activities.

Ab Roll-up

Work your abs in this dancer-friendly version of a crunch.

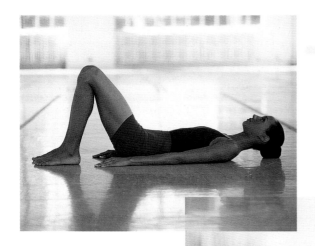

1

Lie on your back with your knees bent and the soles of your feet on the floor near your buttocks. Your arms should extend forward, parallel to your thighs.

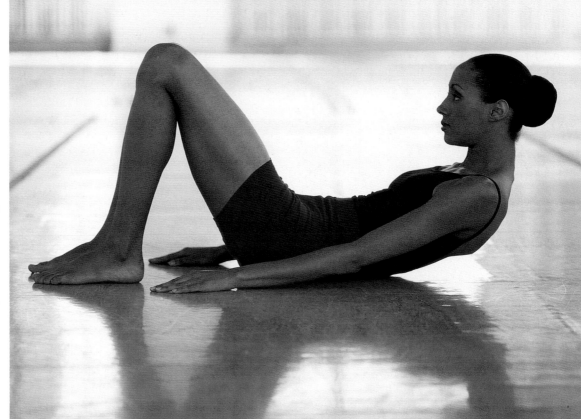

2

Inhale, then exhale as you press your stomach muscles toward your spine and slowly lift your torso up from your abs, rounding your back and neck. You are creating a semicircle with your abdominals as you roll up. Inhale as you slowly curl down, vertebra by vertebra, releasing the tension in your shoulders and neck. Keep reaching forward as you roll. Repeat the Ab Roll-up four to six times.

It's All in Your Mind

The way you visualize movement has a profound effect on its execution. Dancers use all sorts of mental images to help them achieve proper line and shape. Thinking of an extended leg as being "straight as an arrow" can make the difference between creating an elegant, energy-filled line that reaches out into space and one that looks and feels stunted. Imagery also comes into play when visualizing an action. They might also imagine sweeping the floor with one foot in order to produce a soft, brushing motion rather than one that is stiff or jerky.

The same idea holds true for actions that might seem to be less visible but are ultimately just as important to proper technique and line. Concentrate on scooping with your abdominal muscles as you work, and you will lengthen and lift your abs and help strengthen your lower back. If you allow these powerful muscles to bunch and distend, you will loose the all-important connection between your abs and your spine—and end up pushing your abs out rather than lifting them up.

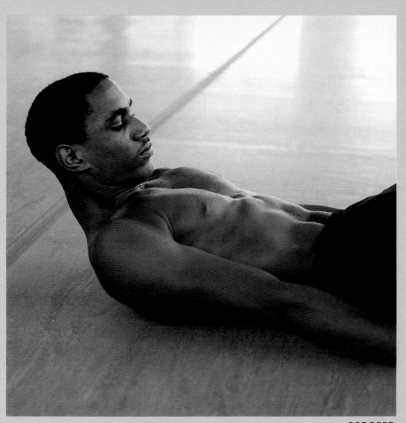

SCOOPED

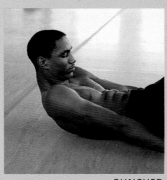

BUNCHED

Ab Pulse

Use the gentle pulsing action of this exercise to activate your abdominals.

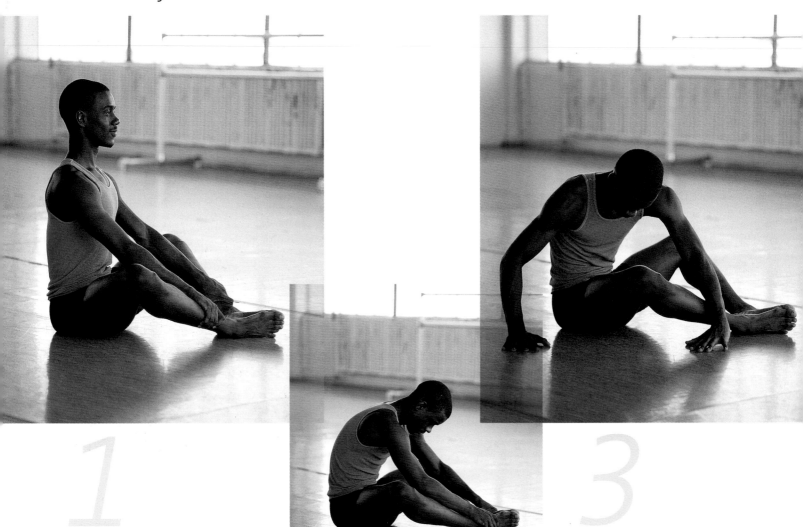

1

Sit upright with the soles of your feet together and your knees open to each side. Your hands should rest on your ankles.

2

Starting with the top of your head, round your back over and toward your feet. Pulse gently eight times in this position. (See page 119.)

3

Turn your torso to your right, place one hand on either side of your right knee, round over, and pulse. Keep both hips on the floor. This position works your obliques (the muscles along the sides of your torso—love handle territory).

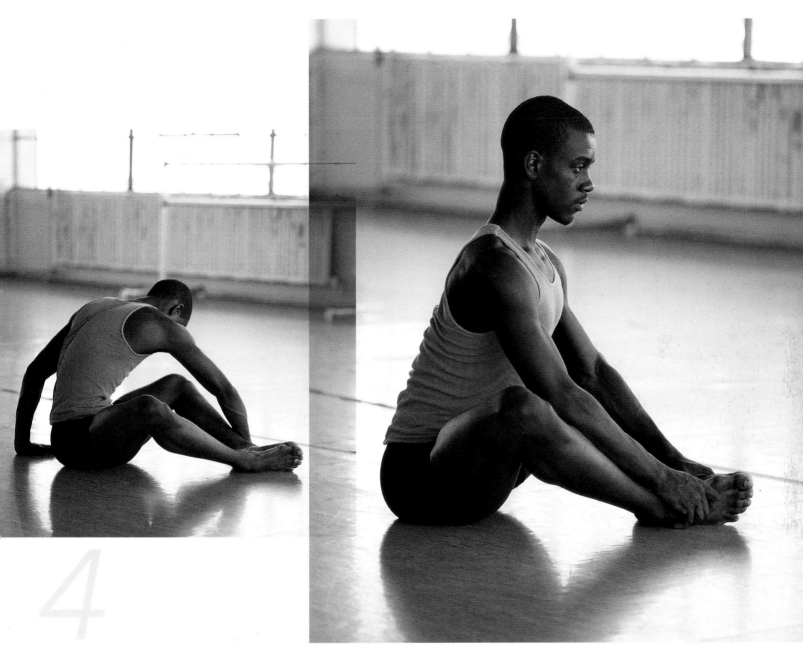

4

Turn your torso to your left and pulse again.

5

Repeat the pulsing action in the center, then starting at the base of your spine, slowly straighten your back so that it creates a long diagonal. Raise your spine upright using the strength of your abdominals.

CONTINUED >

Ab Pulse

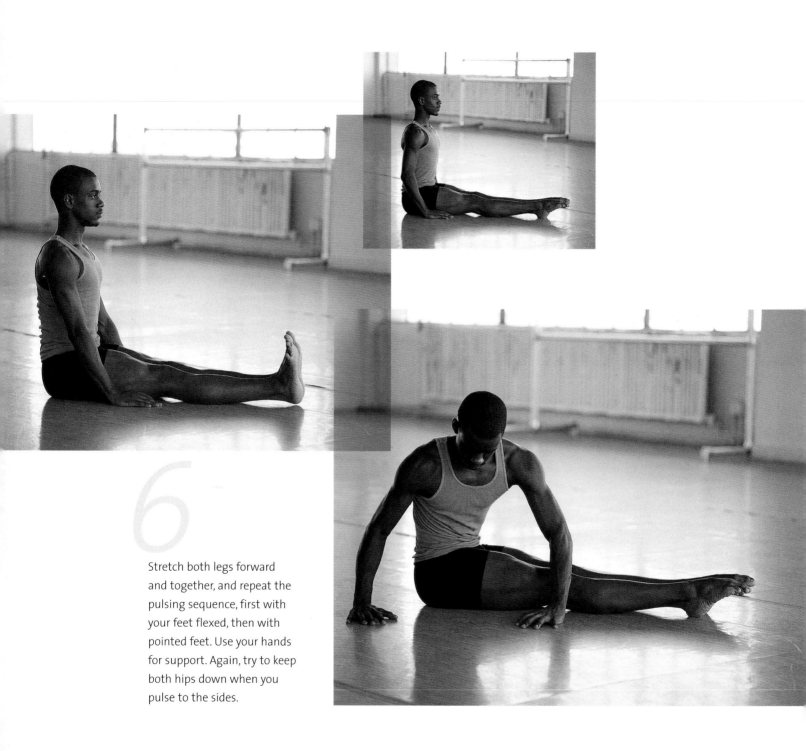

6

Stretch both legs forward and together, and repeat the pulsing sequence, first with your feet flexed, then with pointed feet. Use your hands for support. Again, try to keep both hips down when you pulse to the sides.

Feel the Pulse

The gentle pulsing or rocking motion called for in the ab pulse (see step 2) helps activate and engage your abdominals as it increases flexibility in your hamstrings and calves and releases tension in your hip joints. Pulsing should not be confused with bouncing, a counterproductive action that tends to put your muscles through a vicious cycle of contracting and stretching and, if done too vigorously, can lead to injury.

Initiate the pulsing in your abdominals and allow your torso and head to follow through with an easy stretching and lifting motion. Keep your movements smooth. You'll find that the rhythmic, rocking movement of the pulsing helps make you aware of your breathing, which is always a good thing.

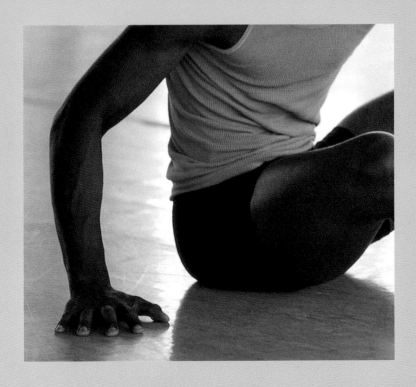

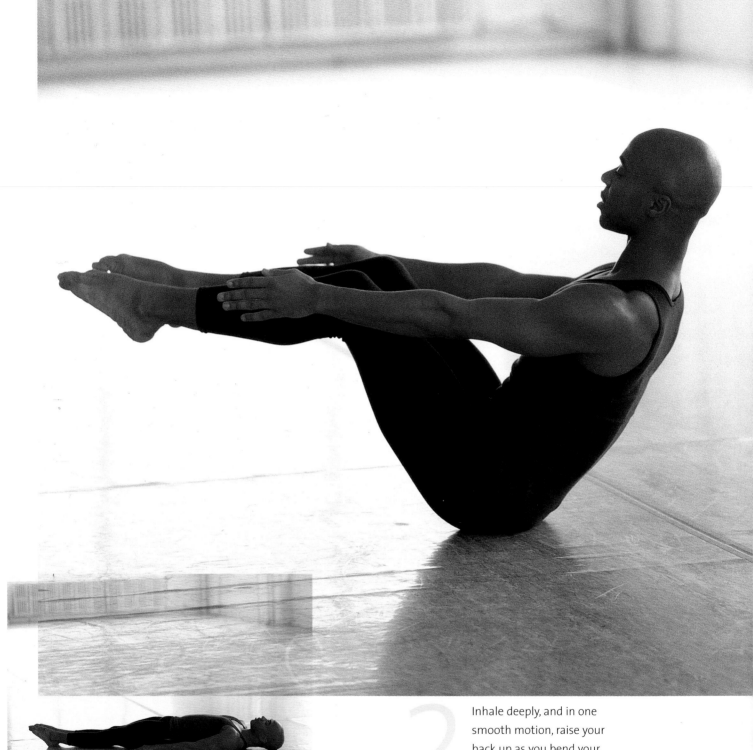

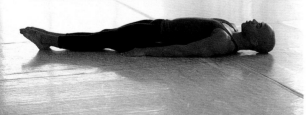

1 Lie on your back with your legs extended and together. Your arms should be along your sides, palms toward the floor.

2 Inhale deeply, and in one smooth motion, raise your back up as you bend your knees and lift your legs off the floor. Your torso and thighs should form a large V shape. Reach your arms forward and try to keep your back as straight as possible.

Teeter-totter

This exercise strengthens your abdominals, back, and quadriceps. You may find it more comfortable if you sit on a folded towel.

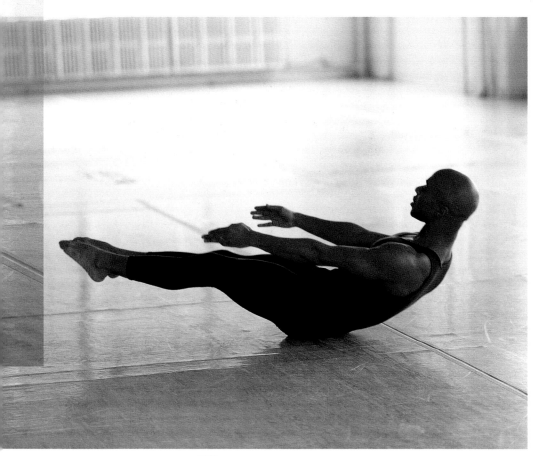

3 Hold this V position for a moment if you can, then exhale as you slowly roll down through your spine and lower your legs.

Repeat the teeter-totter three to six more times.

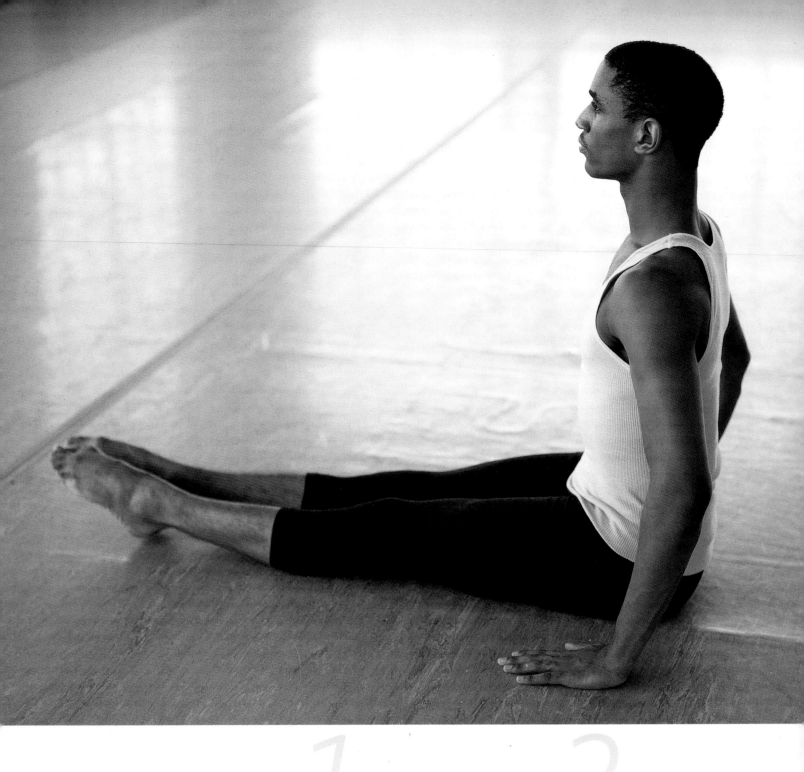

1

Sit with your legs stretched forward and together. Your toes should be pointed and your hands should rest lightly on the floor at your sides. Squeeze your gluteals hard and hold the squeeze for four slow counts.

2

Relax. Repeat six times. Don't be surprised if the squeezing action lifts your heels slightly off the floor.

Gluteal Squeeze

Strengthen and firm your gluteals, a.k.a. your buttocks, with this exercise.

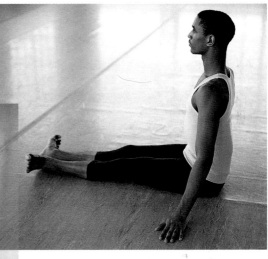

4

Now rotate your legs outward from the tops of your thighs and repeat the exercise. As you squeeze, think of pulling the insides of your thighs upward.

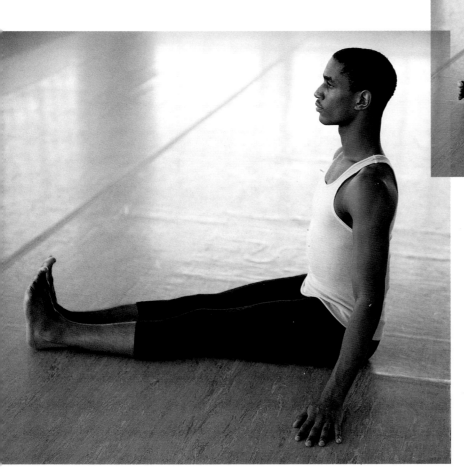

3

Next, repeat the exercise with your feet flexed and together.

Inclined Push-up

If executed with care and concentration, this modified push-up is a wonderful strengthening exercise. You will need a folded towel or small pillow.

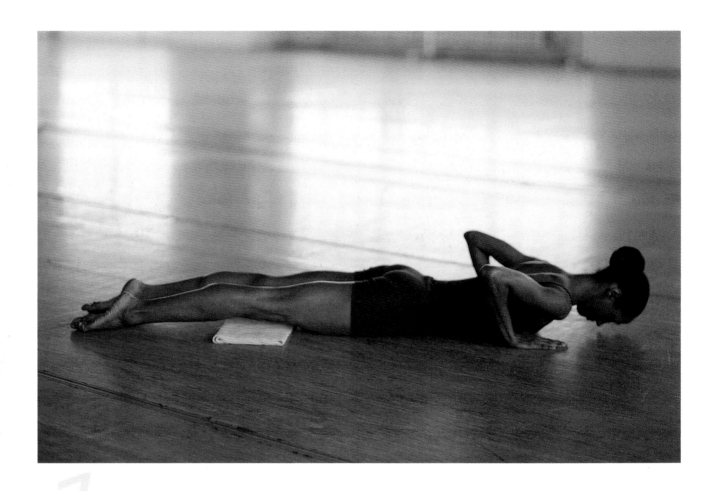

1

Lie on your front with a folded towel or small pillow beneath your knees. Place your hands on the floor next to your shoulders and inhale.

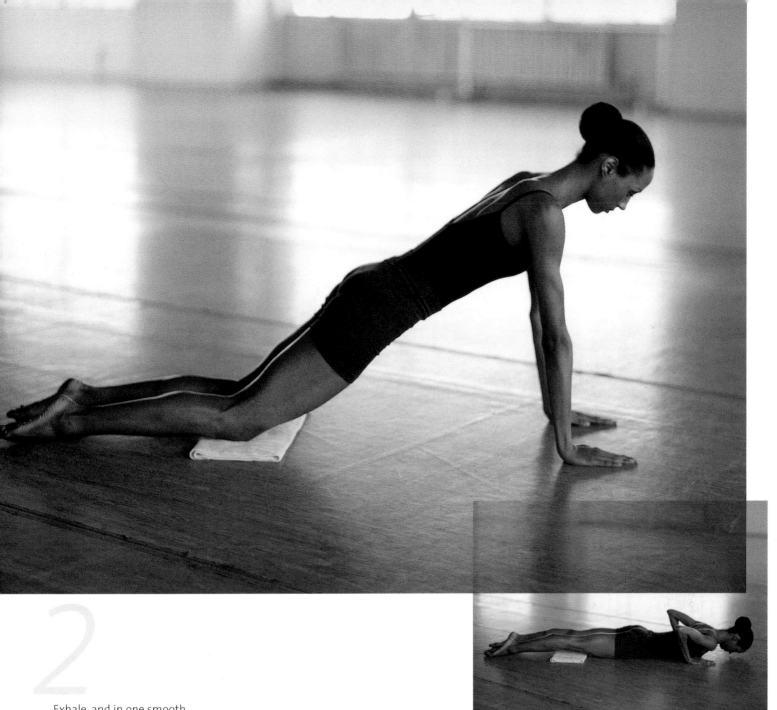

2

Exhale, and in one smooth
motion, press your hands
into the floor and push your
torso up until your elbows are
straight. Your thighs, hips, torso,
neck, and head should form a
diagonal line, from your knees
through the top of your head.

3

Inhale as you lower your torso.
Don't break the line at your
hips or allow your torso to
crumple as you lower.

Repeat the inclined push-up five or
six times.

Heel Slide

This exercise strengthens your hips, hamstrings, and ankles. Be sure to keep both hips on the floor at all times.

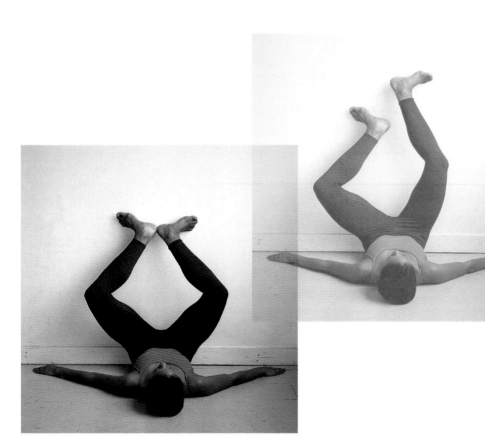

1

Lie on your back with your buttocks flush against the wall and your arms resting comfortably at your sides. Your legs should be bent into a triangle; your feet should be flexed, heels together.

2

Keeping your back and neck long, slowly extend your right leg up the wall, leading with your heel. Your leg should be rotating outward from the top of your thigh.

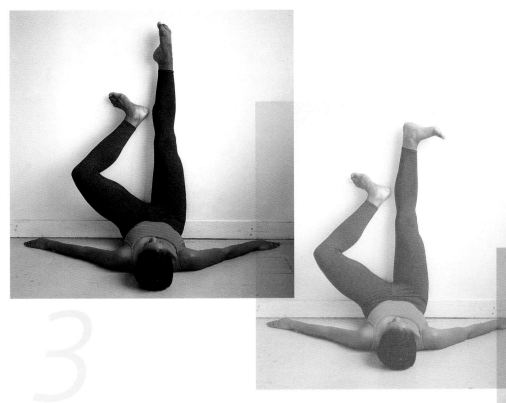

3

When your leg is fully stretched,
point then flex your foot.

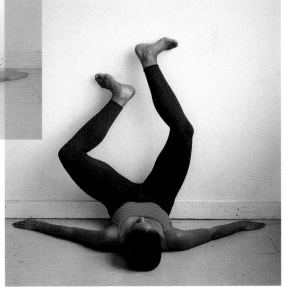

4

Slowly slide your flexed foot
back to the starting position.

Repeat the heel slide with your left
leg, then alternate four times. Try to
keep your abdominals and back long
and strong.

CONTINUED >

Heel Slide

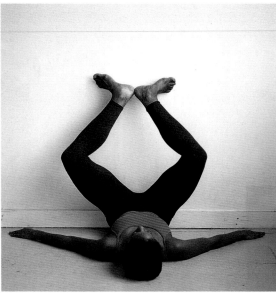

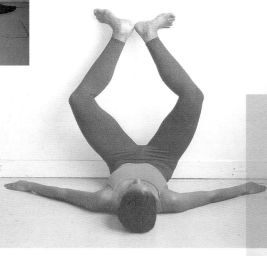

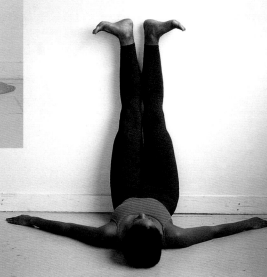

5

Next, try the exercise two to three more times, stretching both legs simultaneously. Try to keep your abdominals and back long and strong.

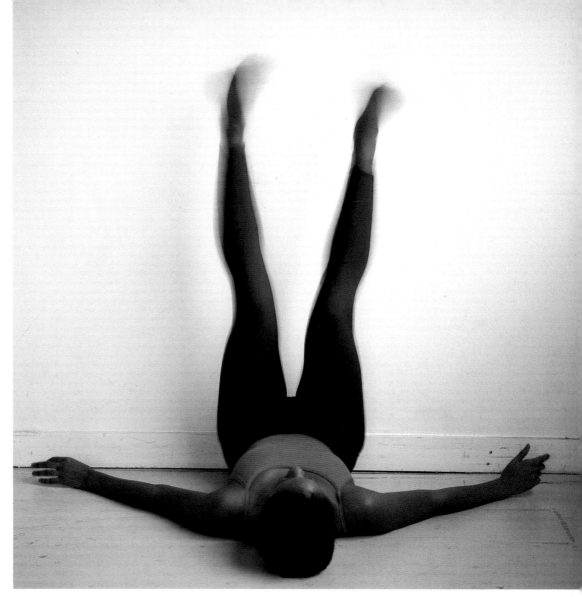

6

Shake out your legs and feet
to release the tension.

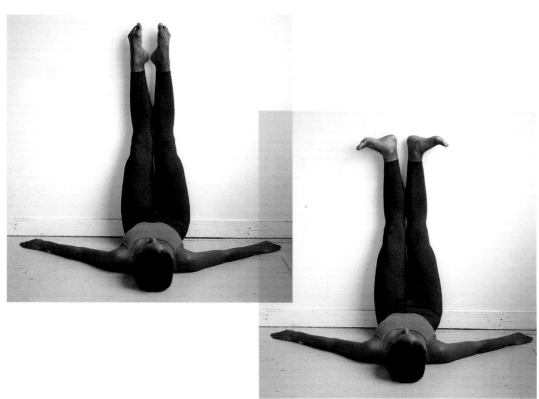

Thigh Press

Use isolation and resistance to increase the strength of your thighs and hips.

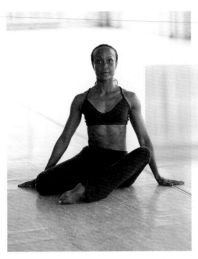

1 Sit upright with your left leg bent so that your shin is parallel to the front of the room and your toes are touching your right knee, which is bent behind you. Your torso should face front and your fingertips should touch the floor.

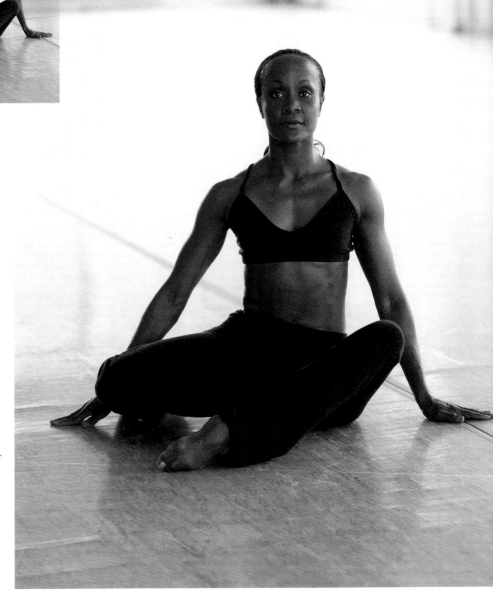

2 Keeping the rest of your body as still as possible, lift your right thigh slightly off the floor in three smooth counts. Your right foot should not move.

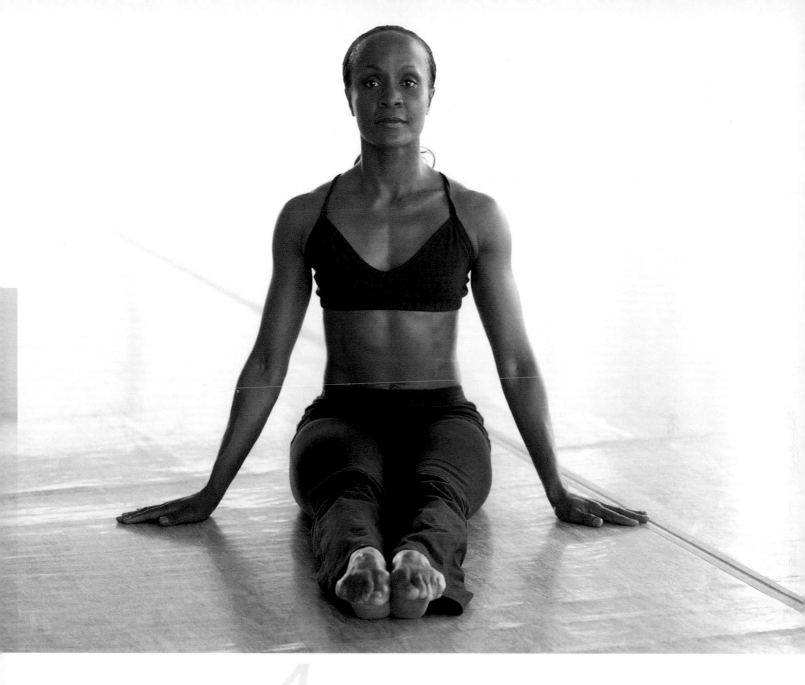

4

Stretch both legs forward then slide into the starting position with your right leg forward this time. You can use your hands for support during the transition.

Repeat the thigh press three times with your left leg.

3

Lower your thigh in three counts, then repeat the thigh press two more times. Don't forget to breathe.

CONTINUED >

Thigh Press

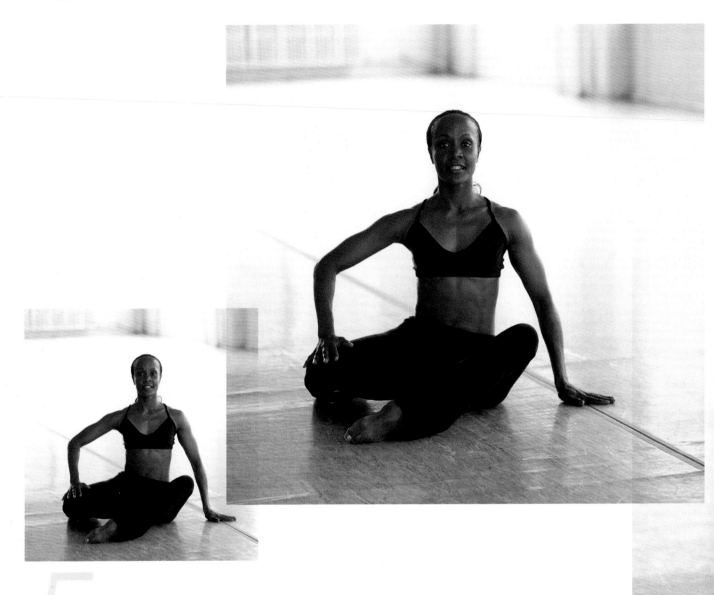

5

Return to your original position, and this time, press down on your right leg with your right hand as you lift. Use your left hand for support. Repeat two more times, increasing the resistance if you wish.

6

Change sides and repeat the thigh press three times with your right leg forward, pressing down on your left thigh. Again, you can increase the resistance with each repetition.

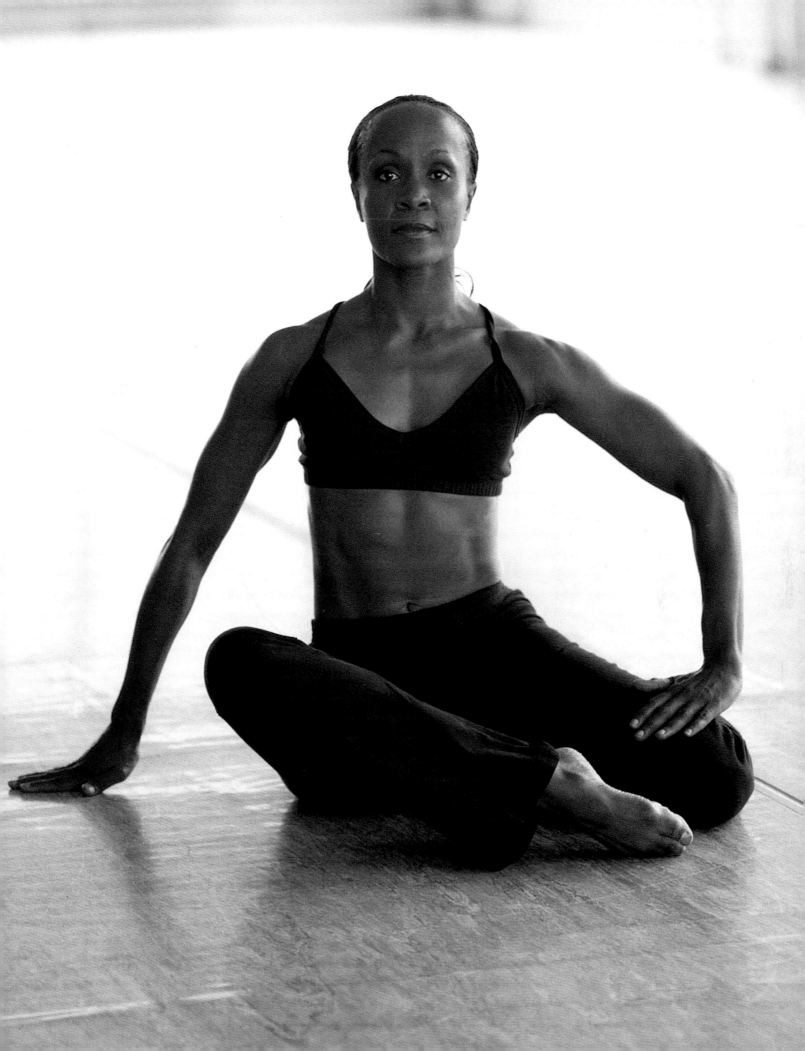

Inner Thigh Lift

Try to keep abdominals and lower back solid as you lift your inner thigh.

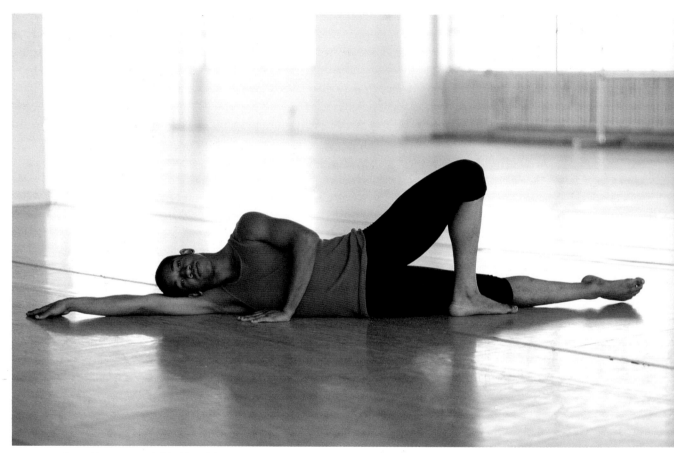

1 Lie on your right side with your right leg extended. Bend your left knee and cross it, placing your left foot on the floor in front of your right thigh. Your left hand should be on the floor near your chest, for support. Your head should rest on your other arm, which is stretched out along the floor.

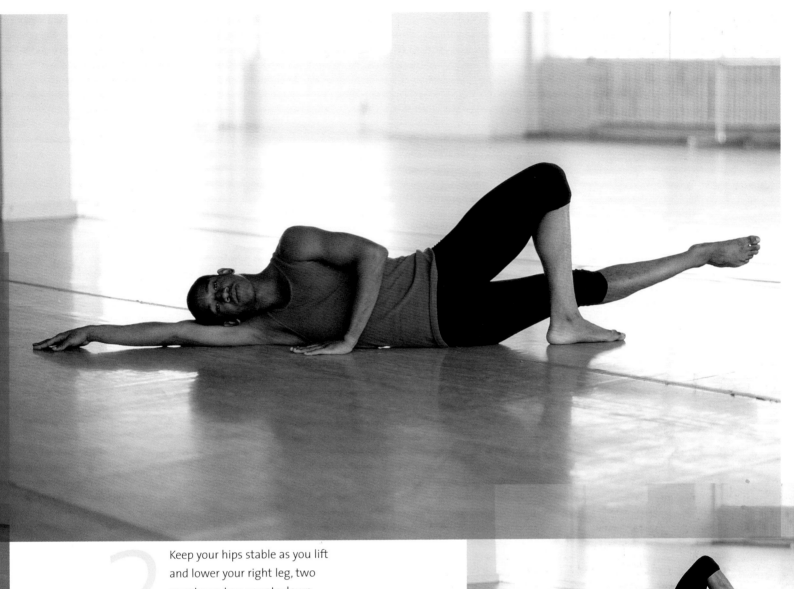

2 Keep your hips stable as you lift and lower your right leg, two counts up, two counts down. Try to keep your leg straight and strong and your abdominals and back long. If you start to roll backward, shift your weight forward slightly, pressing on the floor with your left hand. Lift and lower your leg six times.

3 To change sides, roll onto your back and then onto your left side. Assume the starting position and repeat.

Repeat the inner-thigh lifts on both sides, two to three times.

Demi Plié

The seemingly simple action of bending and straightening your knees yields impressive results when executed with care and attention. As you plié, feel your body lengthening, as if you had a string attached to the top of your head pulling you upward.

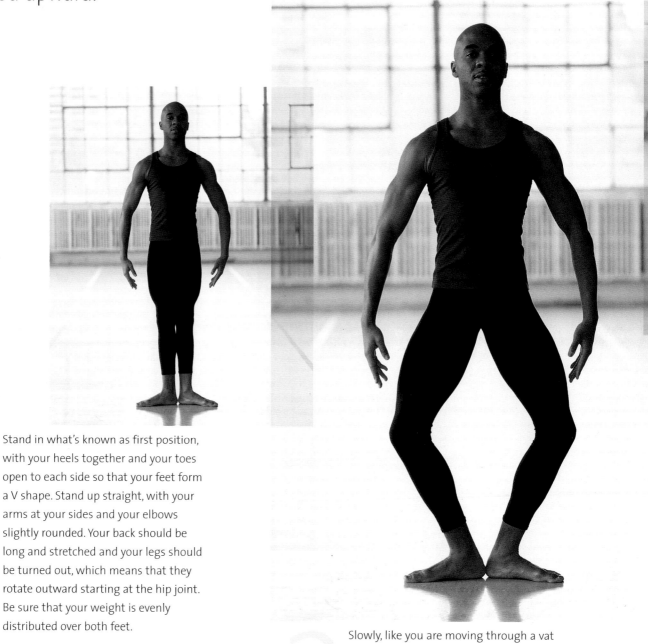

1 Stand in what's known as first position, with your heels together and your toes open to each side so that your feet form a V shape. Stand up straight, with your arms at your sides and your elbows slightly rounded. Your back should be long and stretched and your legs should be turned out, which means that they rotate outward starting at the hip joint. Be sure that your weight is evenly distributed over both feet.

2 Slowly, like you are moving through a vat of honey, bend your knees over your toes, maintaining the outward rotation in your hip joints. Your entire foot should stay on the floor. If your heels start to lift, you're bending too far.

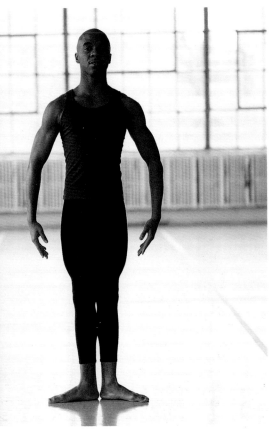

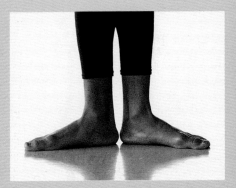

Turnout

"Turning out" the legs may seem like a fairly esoteric concept to nondancers. Yet the same outward rotating action that creates a beautiful line onstage—and enables dancers to move with accuracy and elegance—helps to strengthen and stretch the muscles of the lower back, hips, legs, and feet.

Turnout starts in the hip joints and progresses down through the thighs, knees, lower legs, ankles, and feet. Don't ever force your turnout. Very few of us have 180-degree rotation of the hips. A 45-degree-angle V shape is perfectly acceptable. Your knees should face the same direction as you toes. If you over-rotate your feet, your ankles and insteps will roll in and you might twist and injure your knees.

3 Slowly straighten your legs, engaging the muscles of your buttocks and inner thighs.

Repeat the demi plié four to six times.

HINT The action of a plié is smooth and continuous: don't sit in the bottom of the bend. Because the demi plié helps release tension in the ankles and feet, you might want to repeat it between the two exercises that follow.

Press and Flick

This exercise helps strengthen your quads and stretch your toes, arches, and insteps. You will feel a stretch that runs along your instep and through the ends of your toes. To maintain your balance, lightly hold onto a chair back or countertop.

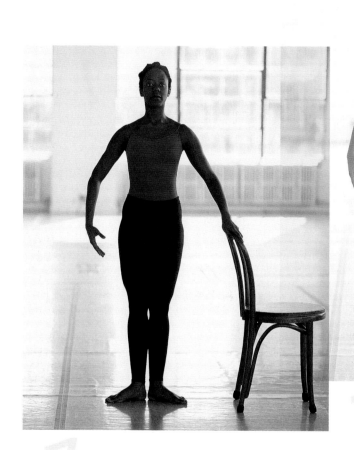

1

Stand in first position. Your back is long and your abdomen is lifted. Your right arm is at your side, elbow slightly rounded.

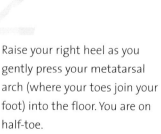

2

Raise your right heel as you gently press your metatarsal arch (where your toes join your foot) into the floor. You are on half-toe.

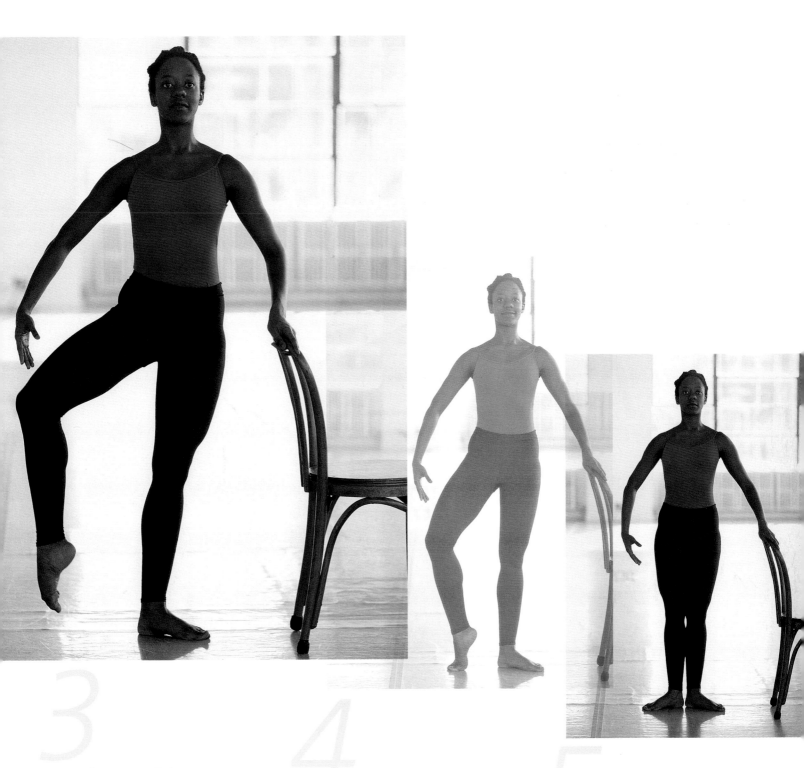

3

From this position, flick your foot until your toes lift off the floor slightly, pointing your toes as they lift. Use the muscles in your toes to push off the floor with a springing action; try not to lift from your knee.

4

Return to the half-toe position, then lower your heel.

5

Do the entire exercise on a count of four: 1. half-toe, 2. flick, 3. half-toe, 4. lower.

Repeat the press-and-flick exercise three or more times on your right foot, then switch to your left.

Tendu and Brush

Tendu, which translates as "stretched," is a ballet exercise that strengthens and stretches your feet. You'll also discover that your buttocks, outer and inner thighs, and calves get a powerful workout from tendu. Use a chair back or countertop to maintain your balance.

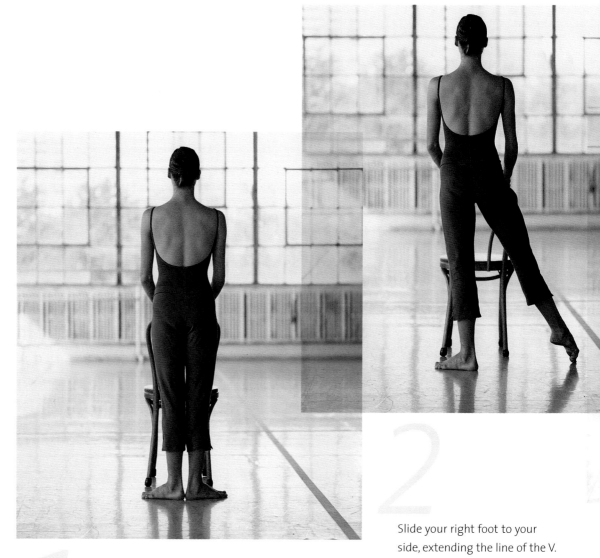

1

Stand in first position.

2

Slide your right foot to your side, extending the line of the V. Lift your heel off the floor as you stretch your foot and point your toes. Feel the muscles working in your arch and the stretch along your instep and through your toes, the tips of which stay in light contact with the floor.

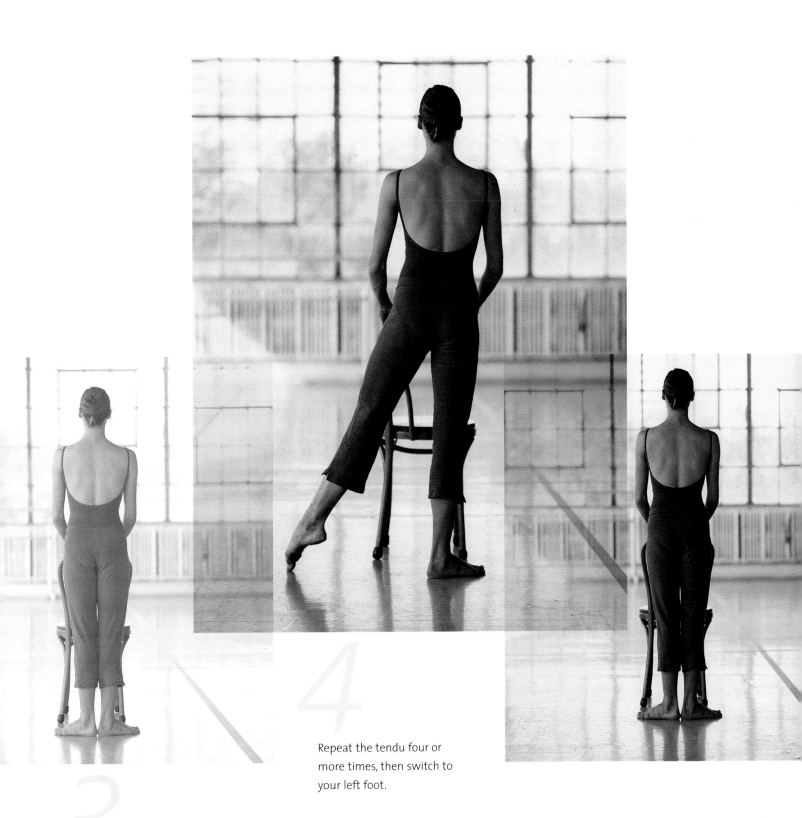

3

Reverse the movement, pulling your foot back until you've closed your heel in first position.

4

Repeat the tendu four or more times, then switch to your left foot.

CONTINUED >

Tendu and Brush

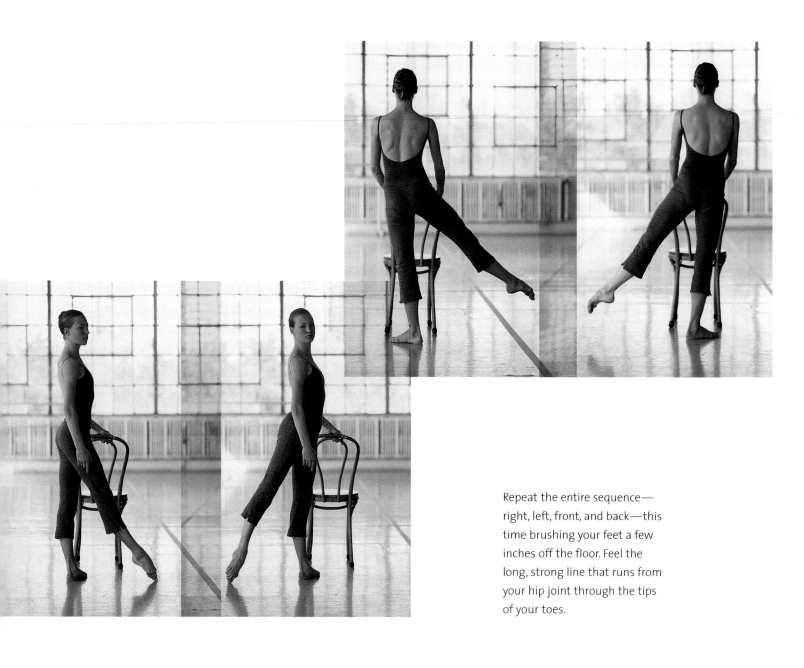

Repeat the entire sequence—
right, left, front, and back—this
time brushing your feet a few
inches off the floor. Feel the
long, strong line that runs from
your hip joint through the tips
of your toes.

Repeat the same movement
four times to the front and four
times to the back with each leg.
Try to keep your torso strong
and your hips still.

Point and Flex

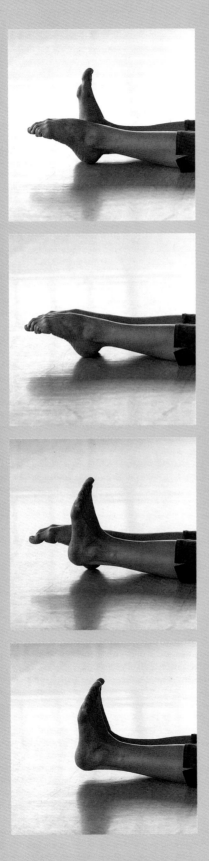

This exercise allows you to concentrate on the fine muscles in your insteps, arches, and toes. Your calves, shins, hamstrings, and quadriceps get into the act as well.

1. Sit on the floor, leaning your back against a wall for support and stretching both legs long in front of you. Your hands should be rested on the floor next to your hips. Be sure that your knees are facing the ceiling.

2. Flex your right foot by pulling your instep and toes back toward your torso as far as you can. Your toes should be pointing straight up. Feel the contraction at the front of your ankle and across your instep and the stretch along your arch.

3. Hold the flex for a moment, then point your toes. Stretch your toes until they're reaching toward the floor. Feel the contraction across the back of your ankle and along your arch, and the stretch along your instep and across the front of your ankle.

Repeat the point-and-flex sequence three more times on your right foot, then switch to your left. Then repeat with both feet at the same time.

I don't let myself get overwhelmed by the full day. I take it in tiny steps.

challenges and rewards

Though it's a challenge to maintain a supple, vibrant body as you get older, the
artistry shines through more. You have life experience to draw from in performance.

For people who have had a troubled background, dancing provides a positive outlet
and a love of beauty, of art.

There's great depth in what we do, and I want to be able to express that to an
audience, to have them leave with something.

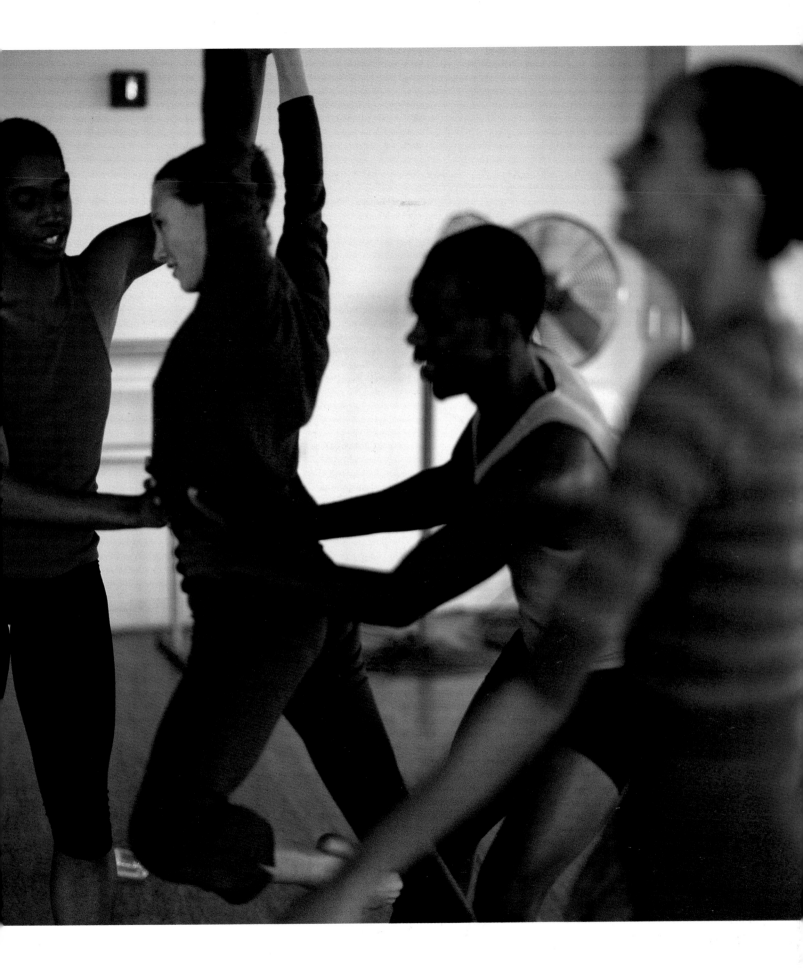

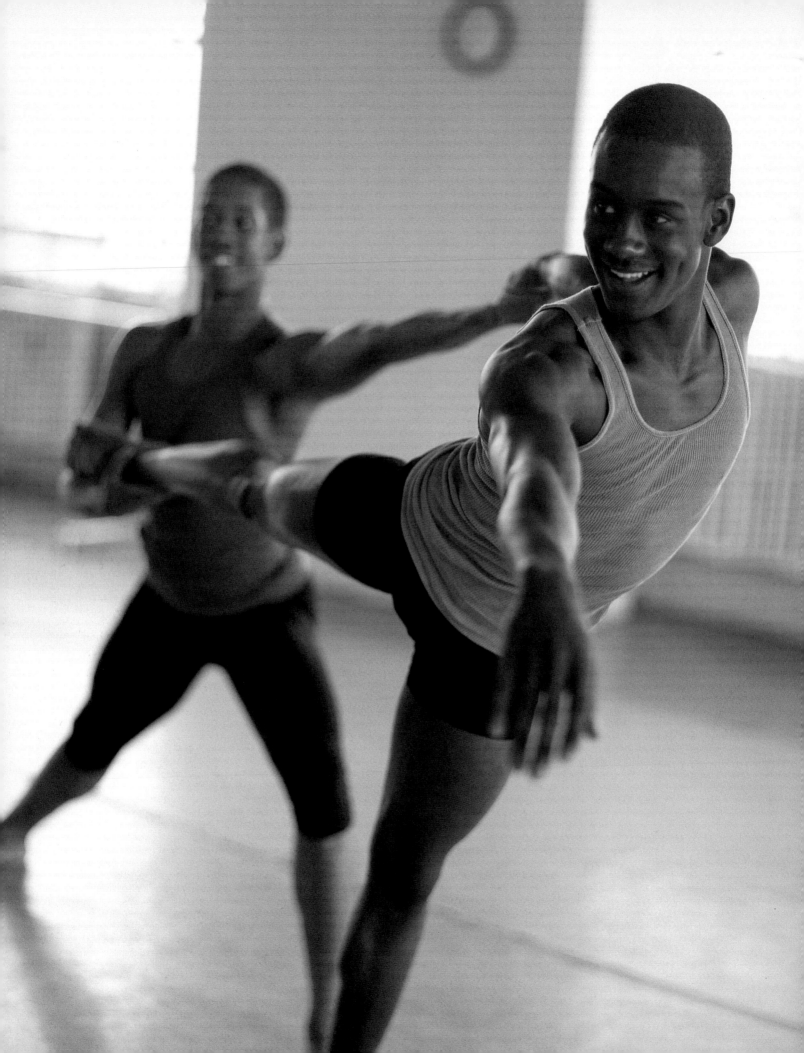

Balance and Coordination

You have devoted care and attention to your warm-up, alignment, stretching, and strengthening exercises. Your body is awake and energized, your mind is fine-focused on the task at hand. It's time to put your pedal to the metal and *move*—every dancer's reason for being!

In this chapter you will encounter exercises to develop your balance and coordination, qualities that enable you to occupy and travel through space with greater awareness, control, and confidence. You will discover how even slight shifts of weight and changes in level and tempo affect your balance. You'll also see how each part of your body works in coordination with another.

Take a walk around the room. The seemingly simple act of placing one foot in front of the other is actually a rich and complex action. Your center of gravity continuously shifts with every step you take. Rise onto half-toe or transfer your base of support from two feet to one, and you've added even more variables to the mix.

You'll also notice how subtle variations in rhythm, scale, and dynamics dramatically influence the impact of a particular exercise. If, for example, you do the Pony (see page 156) at an extremely slow tempo, then repeat it at twice the speed, you will find that you emphasize—and reveal—entirely different aspects of the same movements. This ability to inhabit and inflect movement with individuality and nuance is one of dancing's greatest rewards.

The Dancer

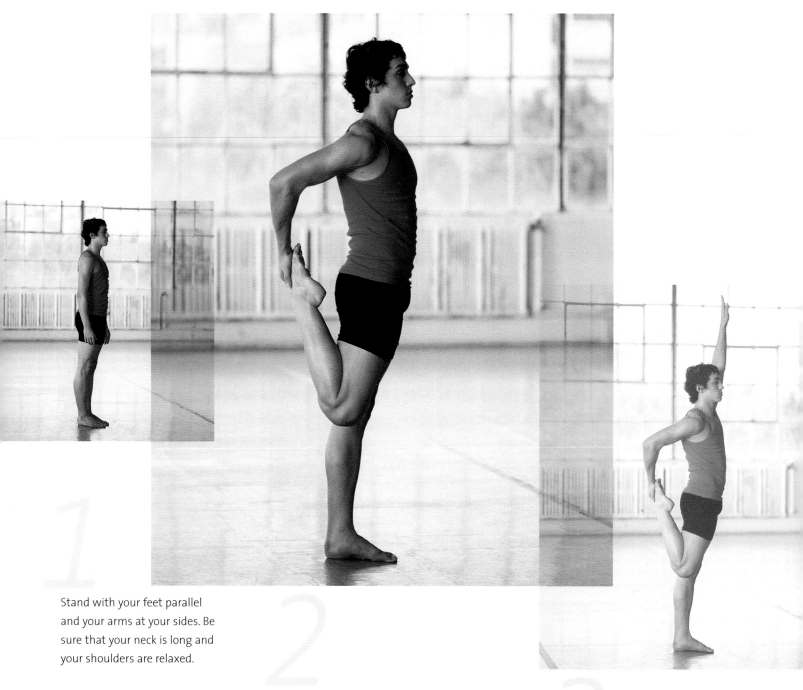

Stand with your feet parallel and your arms at your sides. Be sure that your neck is long and your shoulders are relaxed.

Shift your weight onto your left foot and bend your right knee slightly. Take a deep breath as you reach back with your right arm and grasp your right foot. Exhale, focusing on a spot on the floor for balance.

Inhale and reach your left hand toward the ceiling.

In addition to providing a great stretch through your hips, legs, back, and shoulders, the Dancer helps improve your balance and concentration. If you like, use a chair back or countertop to help maintain your balance.

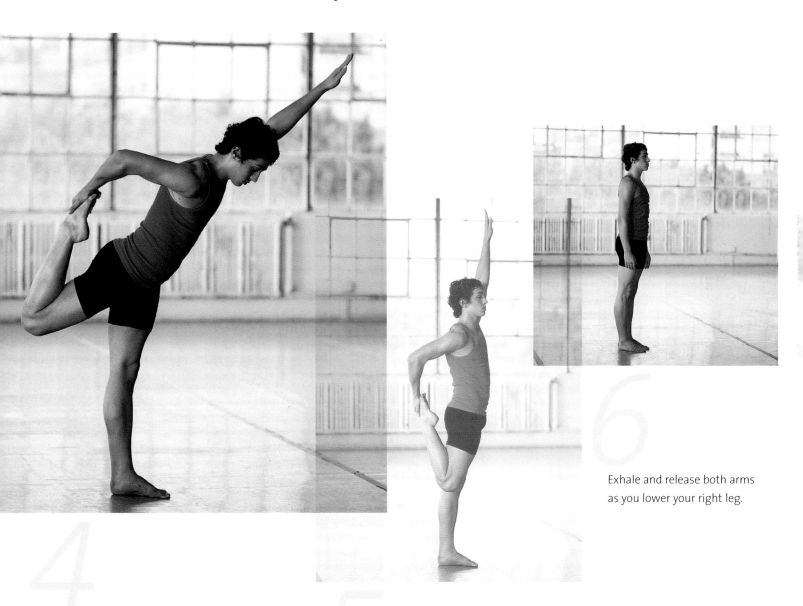

Exhale and release both arms as you lower your right leg.

Exhale and lift your right leg higher behind you, still firmly holding onto your foot. As you lift, tilt your torso forward from your hips. Keep your back straight, and try to keep both hips parallel to the floor. Try to hold this position for a few deep breaths.

Inhale and lift your left arm overhead, at the same time bringing your torso upright. Your torso is like a lever.

Repeat the Dancer on the left side. If you have trouble balancing, take your time—it's a bit tricky. Try it in stages until you feel confident and secure.

Balancing Act

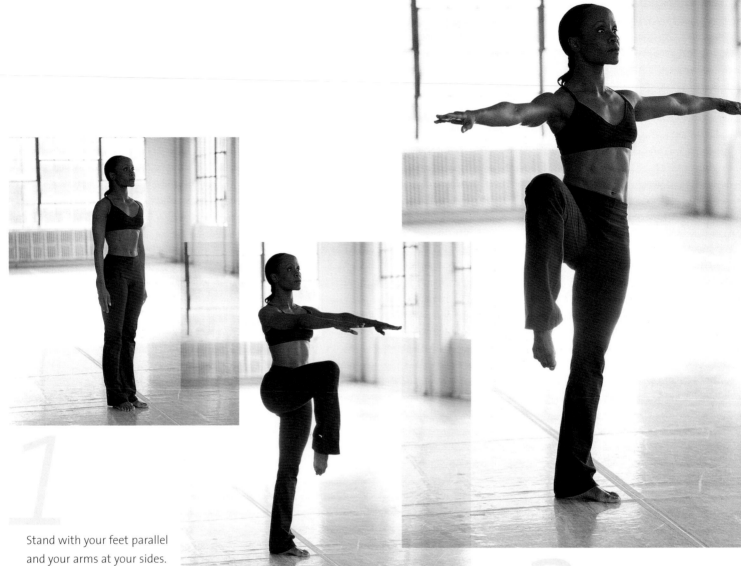

Stand with your feet parallel and your arms at your sides.

Raise your arms forward to chest height as you lift your right knee; ideally, your thigh should be parallel to the ceiling. If this is too difficult, aim for a 45-degree angle.

Slowly and smoothly, open your arms to your sides as you open your right leg to the side. Imagine you are opening a curtain with your arms. Try to keep your left leg and back long and strong.

Strong abdominals and a lifted torso help you find and maintain your balance in this exercise. If you feel wobbly, you can hold onto the back of a chair or countertop with one hand for support, but, as you gain confidence, try the exercise hands-free.

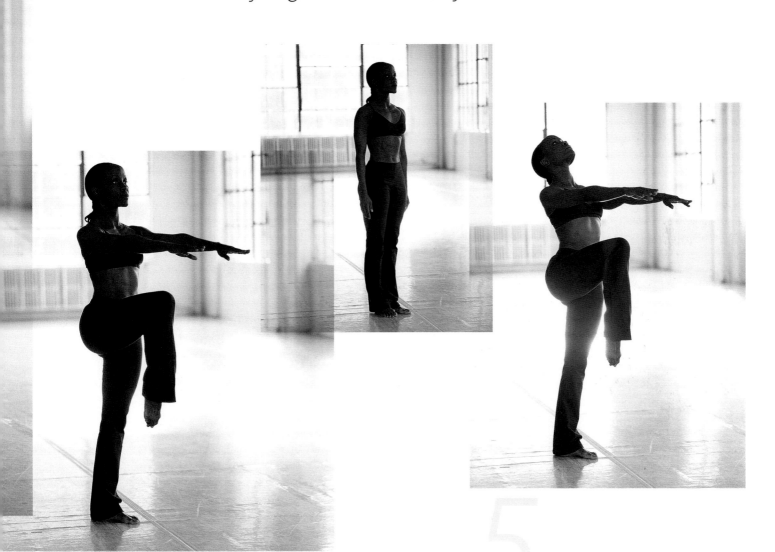

4

Bring your arms and knee back to the center position. Your hips should be level. Lower your arms and leg to the starting position.

5

Repeat Balancing Act on the left side. If your balance is spot-on, try adding a small arch of the upper back at step 4 on both sides.

Box Step

In this exercise, you'll be "drawing" two side-by-side boxes with your feet. This helps you learn the dancer's task: to make patterns as you move through space.

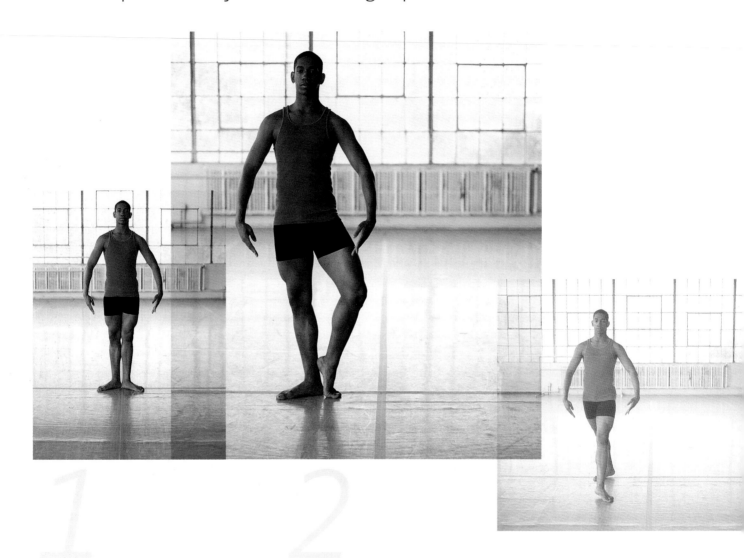

Stand in first position, with your heels together and your toes open to a 45-degree angle. Your arms should be at your sides and slightly rounded.

Step sideways with your right foot and bring your left toes to your right heel.

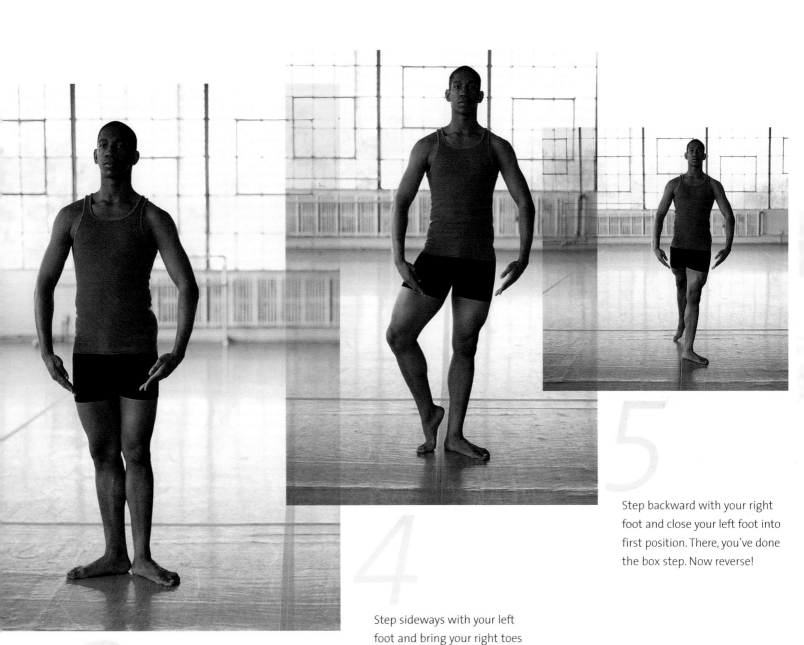

5

Step backward with your right foot and close your left foot into first position. There, you've done the box step. Now reverse!

4

Step sideways with your left foot and bring your right toes to your left heel.

3

Step forward with your left foot and close your right foot into first position.

HINT Looking at the dancer's position relative to the intersecting lines on the floor will help you see the pattern.

CONTINUED >

Box Step

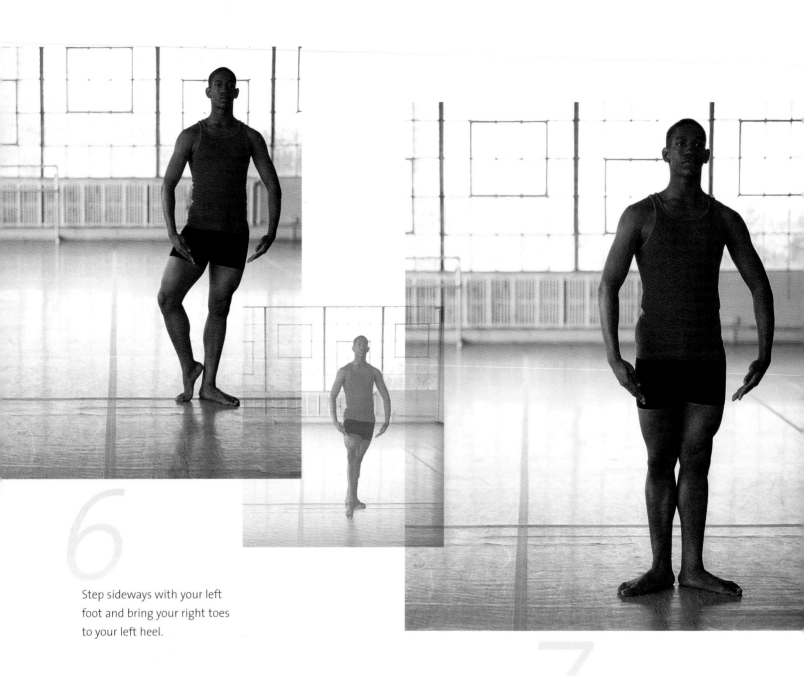

6 Step sideways with your left foot and bring your right toes to your left heel.

7 Step forward with your right foot and close your left foot into first position.

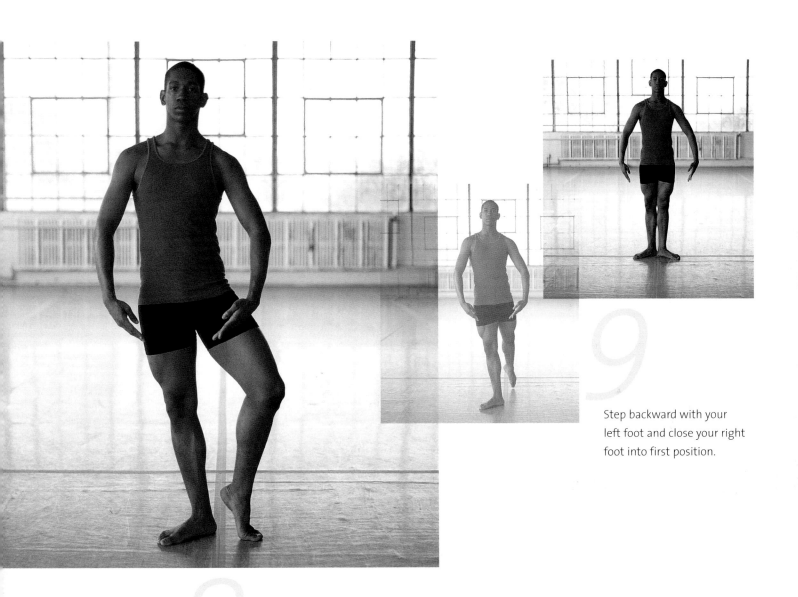

9

Step backward with your left foot and close your right foot into first position.

8

Step sideways with your right foot and bring your left toes to your right heel.

You'll feel the natural rhythm of the Box Step if you take large, full steps. Use each step to create a clear pattern on the floor. The movement might feel even more expansive if you hold your arms open to the side. Feel free to play with the tempo as you become comfortable with the pattern.

Do the Pony

The natural springing action of this prancing exercise propels you from side to side. Think of a horse's delicate, well-defined legs and hooves as you increase the dimension and scope of your movements.

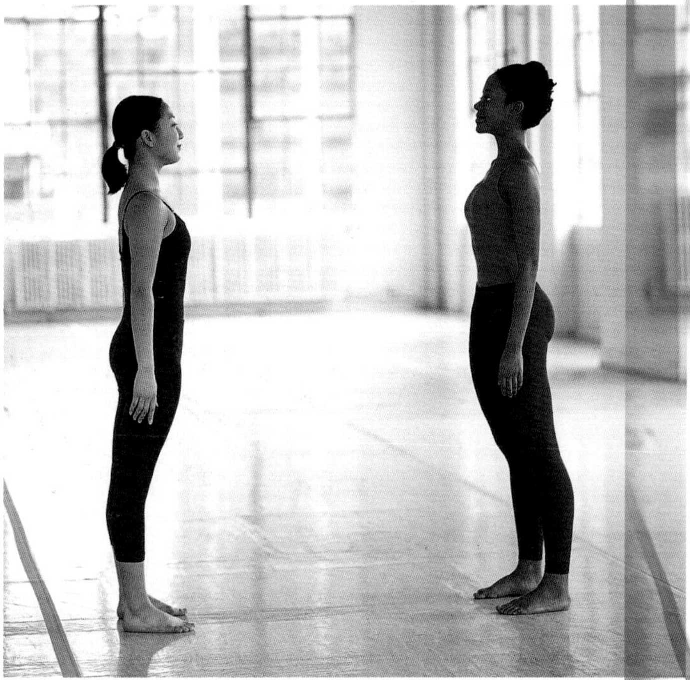

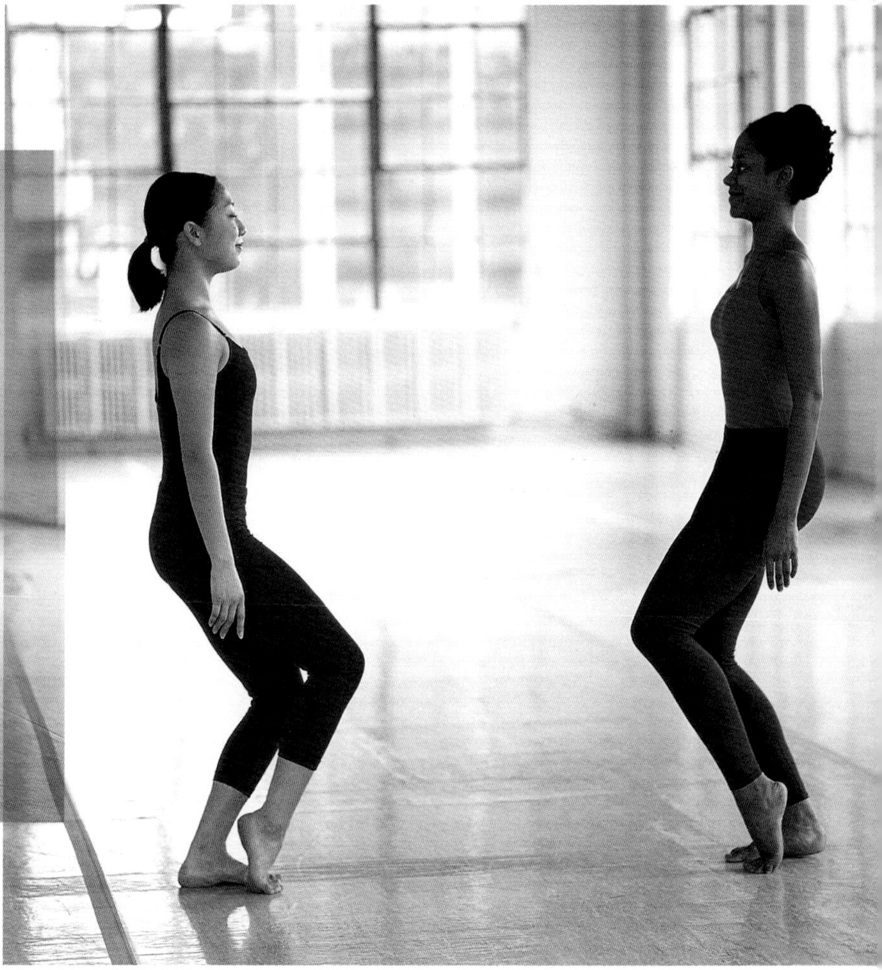

1

Stand with your feet parallel and your arms hanging at your sides.

2

Plié on both legs, then push off the floor with the balls of your feet, transferring your weight onto your right foot and lifting your left foot slightly off the floor. Your left knee should be lifted to the front.

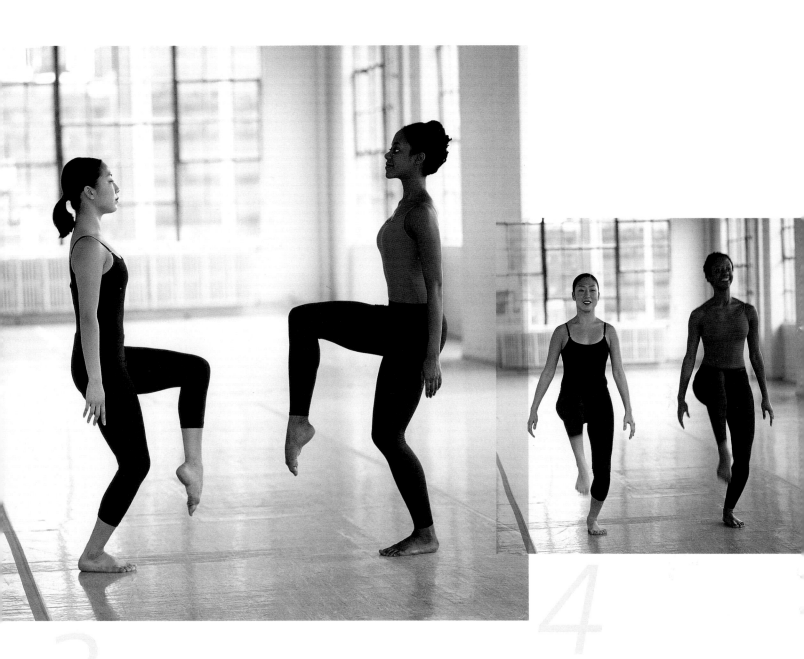

3

Repeat the prance, transferring
your weight onto your left foot.
Keep your abdomen lifted.

4

Alternate sides several times,
establishing an easy, loping
rhythm.

The rhythm is prance-and-tap; prance-
and-tap; ya-da-*da*, ya-da-*da*. Play with
the tempo and the size of the Pony.

CONTINUED >

Do the Pony

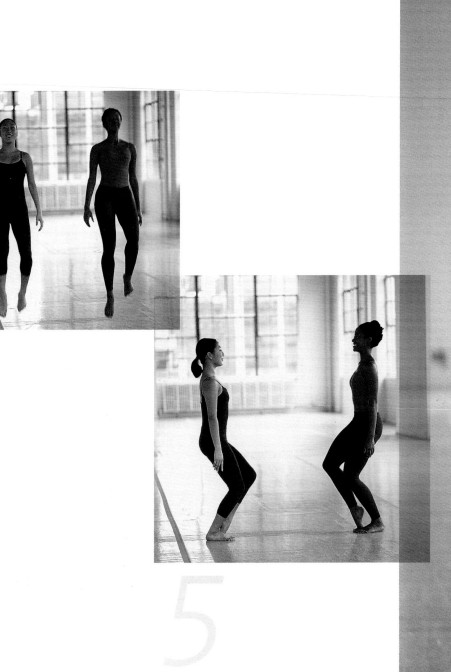

5

Now add a small tap of the foot. If you ever done the popular dance called the Pony, you've got it. Prance onto your right foot and tap the toe of your left foot on the floor.

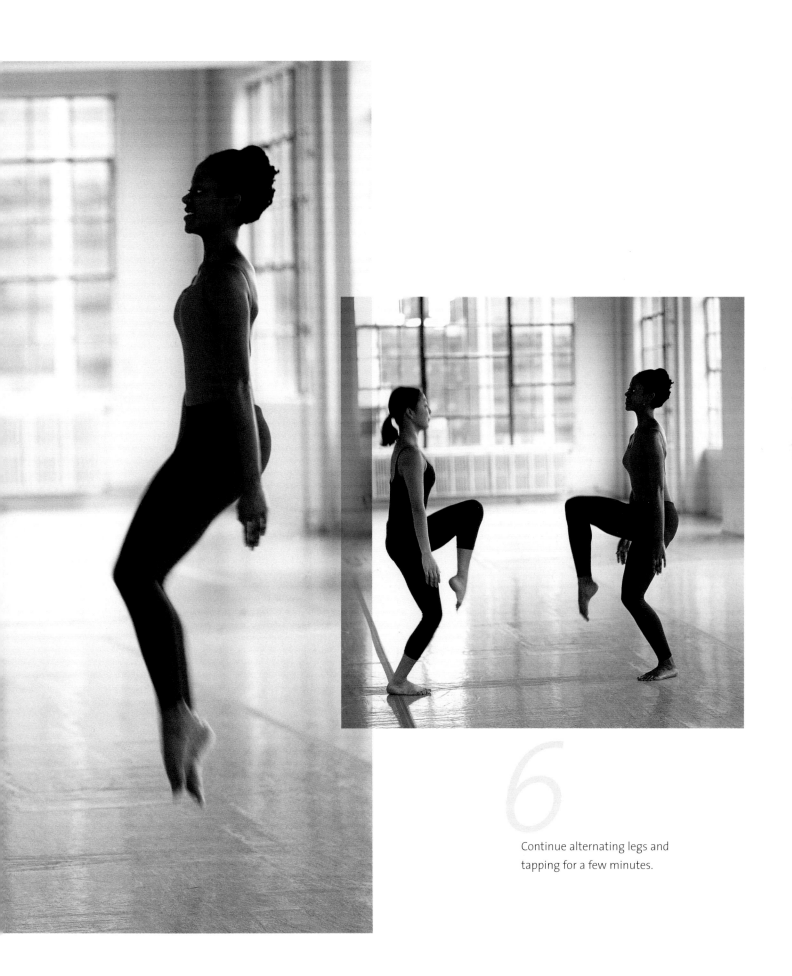

6

Continue alternating legs and tapping for a few minutes.

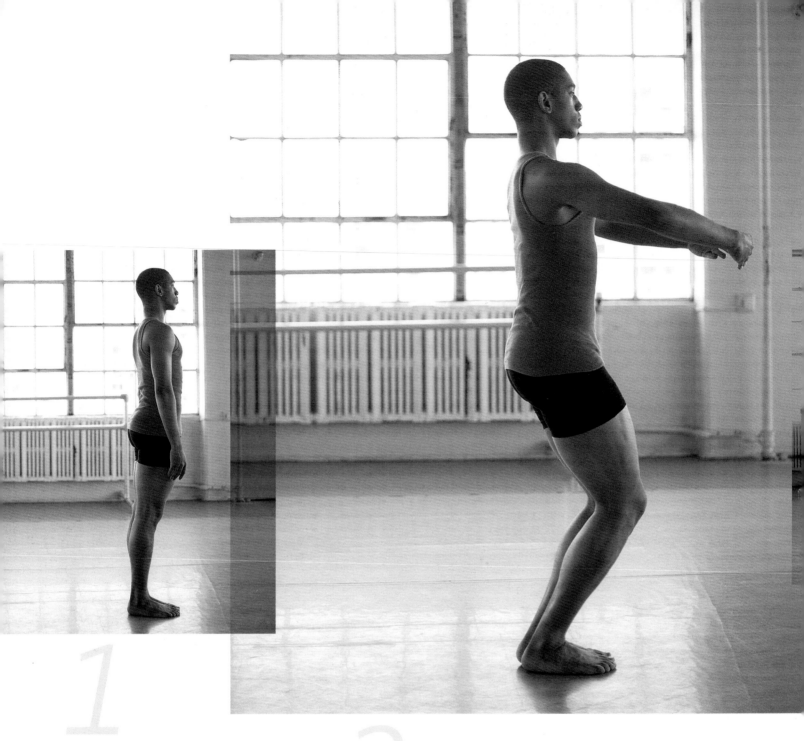

1

Stand with your feet parallel,
your arms at your sides.

2

Plié on both legs as you round
your arms and bring them
forward, in front of your chest.

Low and Loose

Keep your weight low and your torso, pelvis, and arms loose. Give in to the natural rhythm of the rebound and you'll find your coordination.

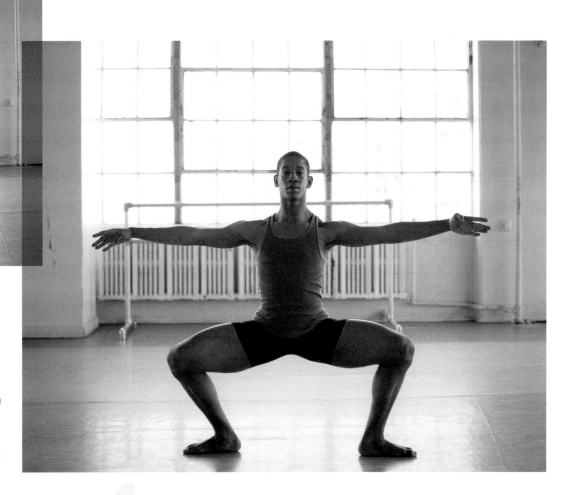

3

Push out of the plié with a springing action as you open your right leg and torso and lift your arms overhead. You are making a quarter turn to the right.

4

Open your arms to your sides and land softly in a plié. Your left foot may shift slightly so it is pointing forward. That will help you keep your balance.

CONTINUED >

Low and Loose

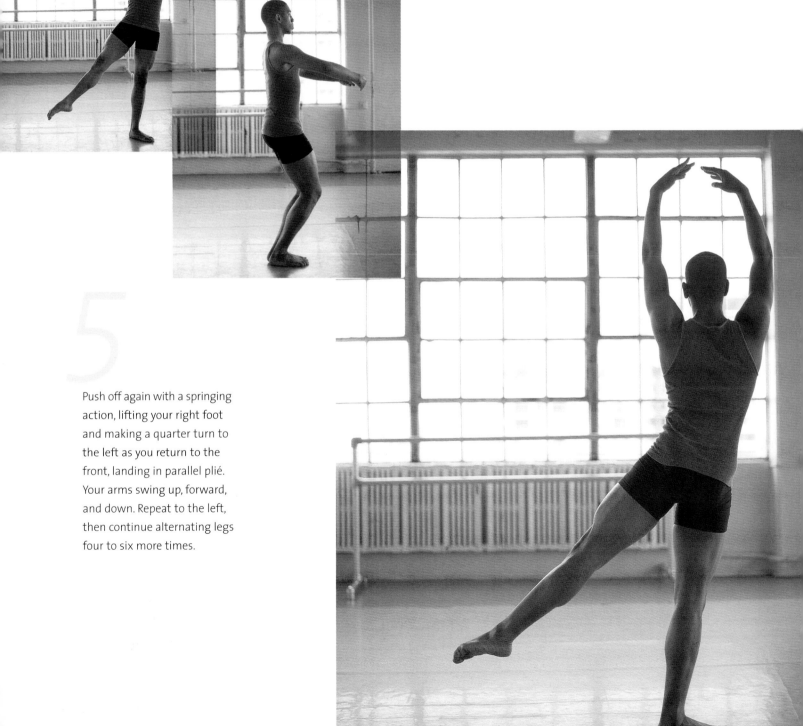

Push off again with a springing
action, lifting your right foot
and making a quarter turn to
the left as you return to the
front, landing in parallel plié.
Your arms swing up, forward,
and down. Repeat to the left,
then continue alternating legs
four to six more times.

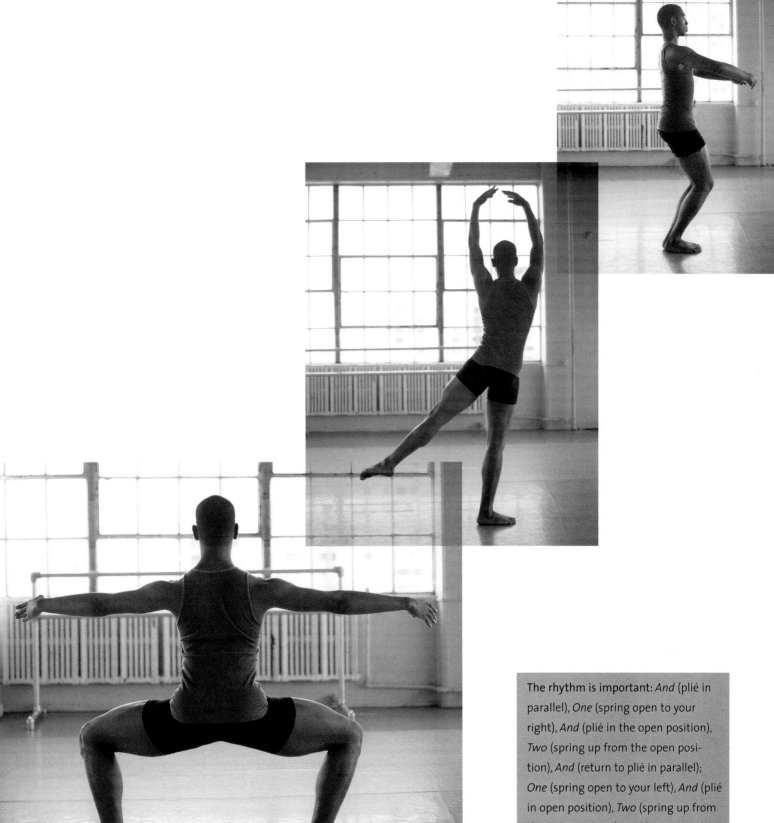

The rhythm is important: *And* (plié in parallel), *One* (spring open to your right), *And* (plié in the open position), *Two* (spring up from the open position), *And* (return to plié in parallel); *One* (spring open to your left), *And* (plié in open position), *Two* (spring up from the open position), *And* (return to plié in parallel).

HINT Play with the tempo and the size of the steps. See how much spring you can get when you push off.

Walk Like an Egyptian

Move your upper and lower body in opposition with this stylized walk.

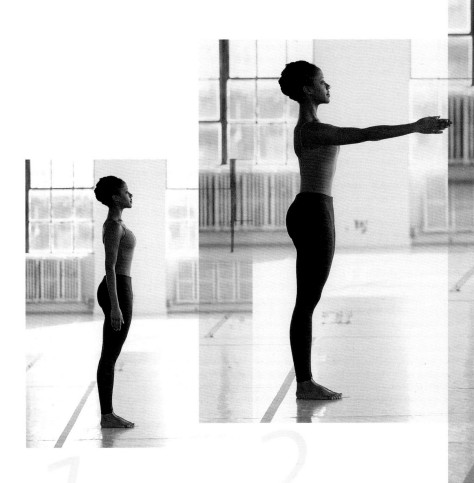

1

Stand in parallel with your arms at your sides.

2

Raise your arms forward up to chest height. Your palms should face each other.

3

Bend your forearms up, so that your elbows form right angles. As you raise your forearms, rotate your palms toward your face.

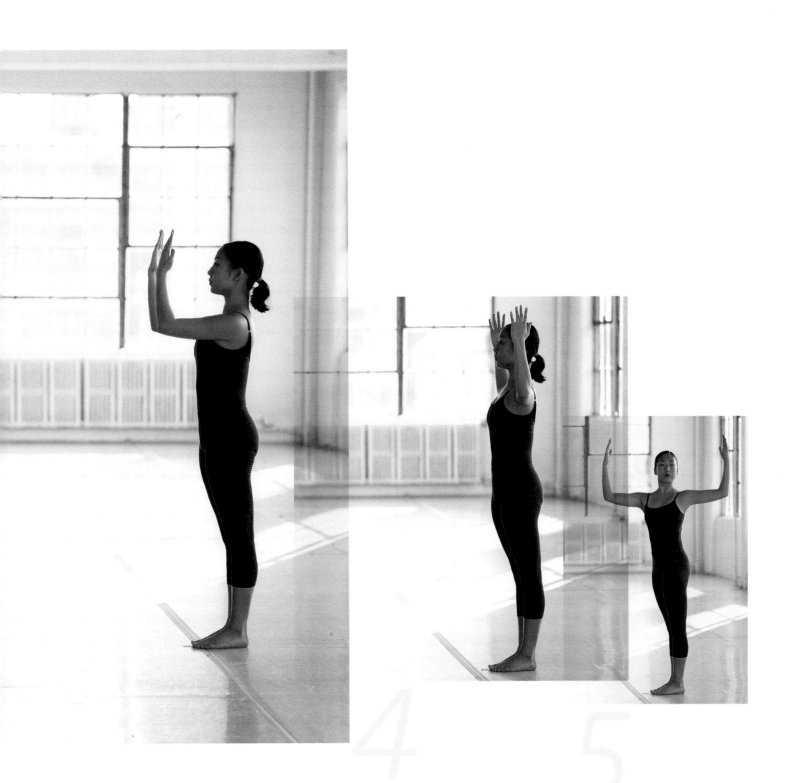

Open your elbows to your sides, making sure to hold on to the shape. If you can't see both arms in your peripheral vision, you've opened them too far.

Now twist your torso, neck, and head to your left, as far as you can while keeping your hips facing front. Your upper body should remain still.

CONTINUED >

Walk Like
an Egyptian

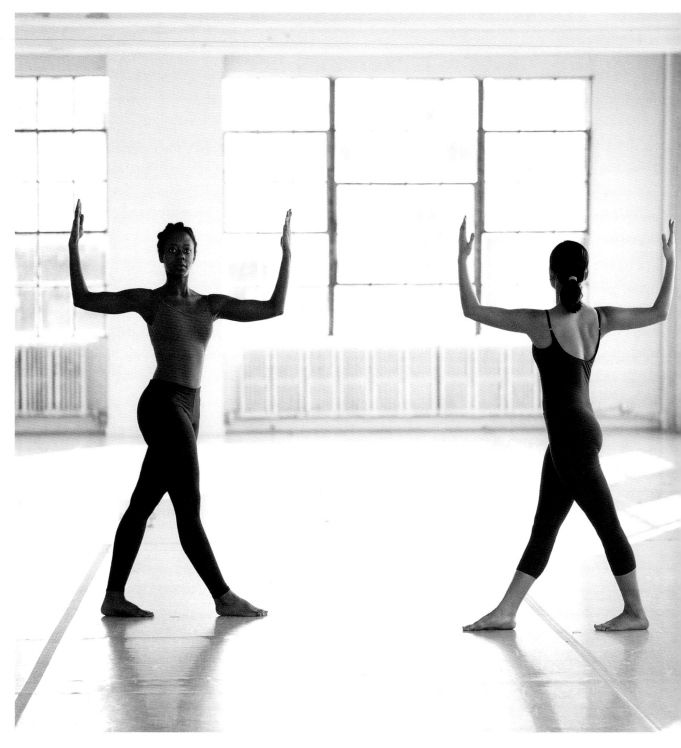

Now twist to your right.

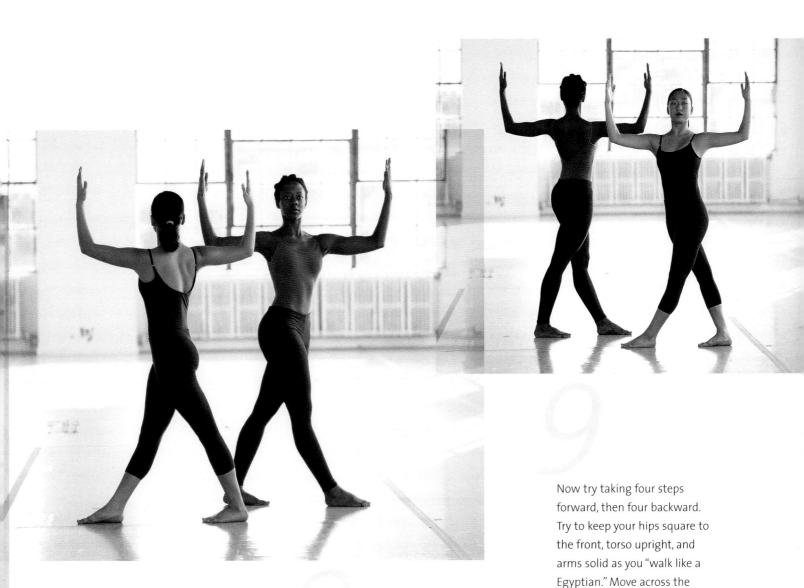

Now try taking four steps forward, then four backward. Try to keep your hips square to the front, torso upright, and arms solid as you "walk like a Egyptian." Move across the room and back.

Twist to the left and step forward with your left foot. Lead with your toes. The twisting action will feel more emphatic and clear if you make your steps brisk and bold.

Repeat the twisting action as you take a step forward. When you twist to the right you step forward with your right foot.

As you do this exercise, think of the elegant figures depicted in Egyptian wall paintings. Their hips face forward as they walk, yet their torsos are swiveled to the side.

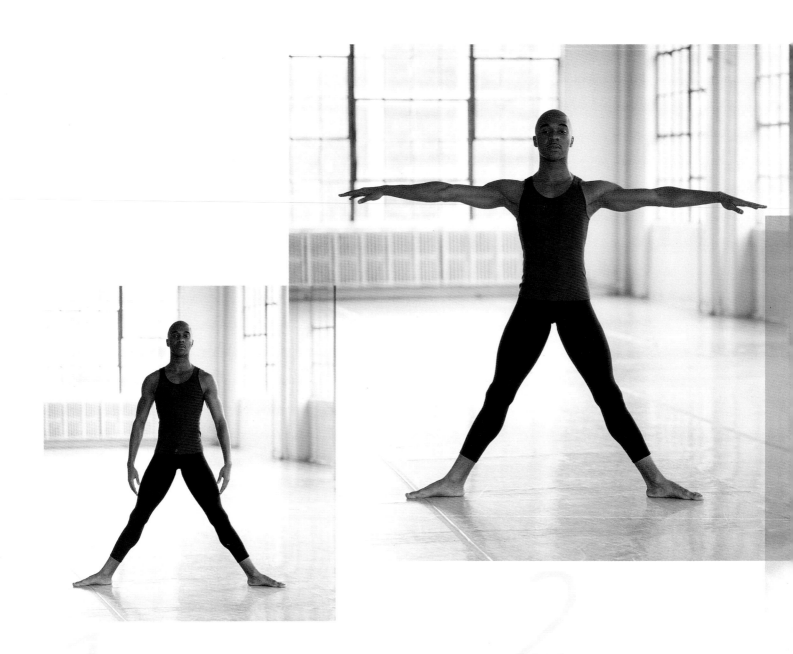

Stand in a wide second
position with your arms
hanging at your sides.

Raise your arms to shoulder
height and lunge into your
right leg, straightening your
left. Both feet should stay firmly
planted on the floor. If you start
to tip over, make your lunge a
little smaller.

Swiveling Lunge

The coordination of the deep lunging action, a mobile torso, and expressive arms make this exercise a power-house. Move slowly and smoothly.

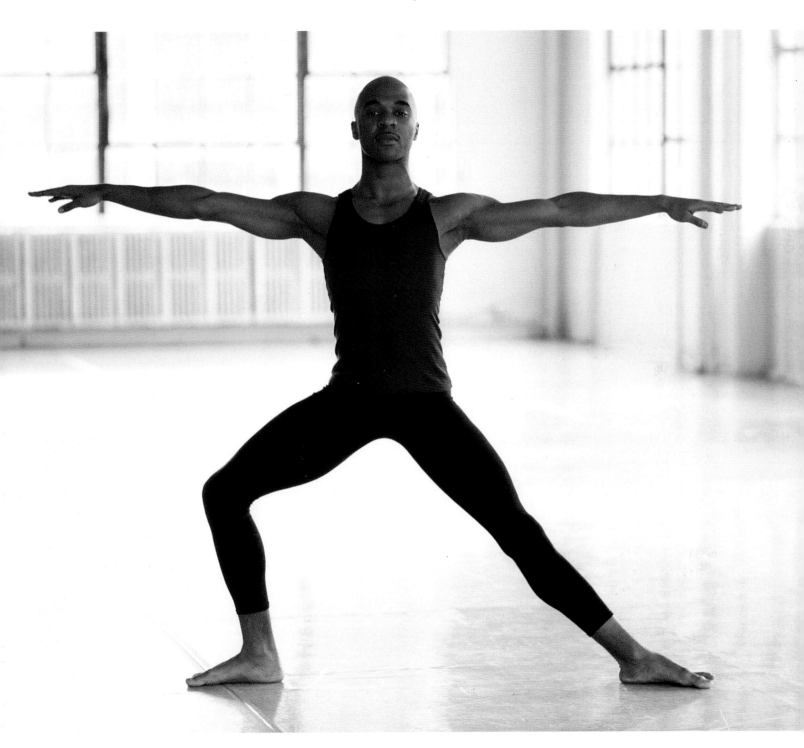

CONTINUED >

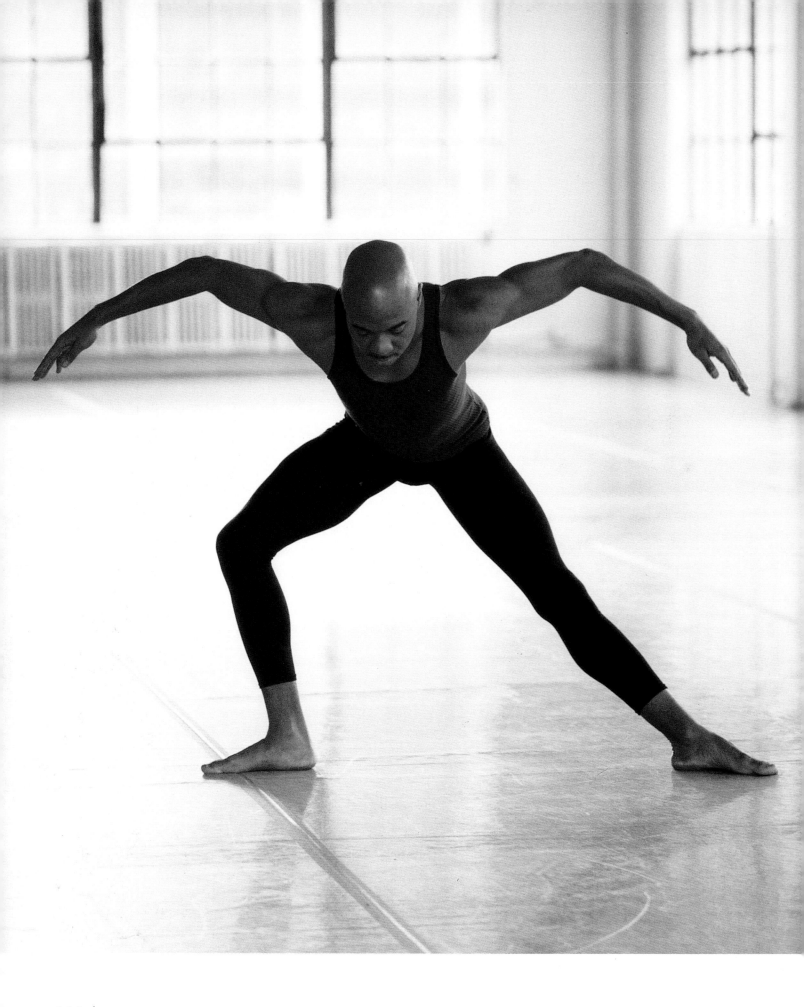

Swiveling Lunge

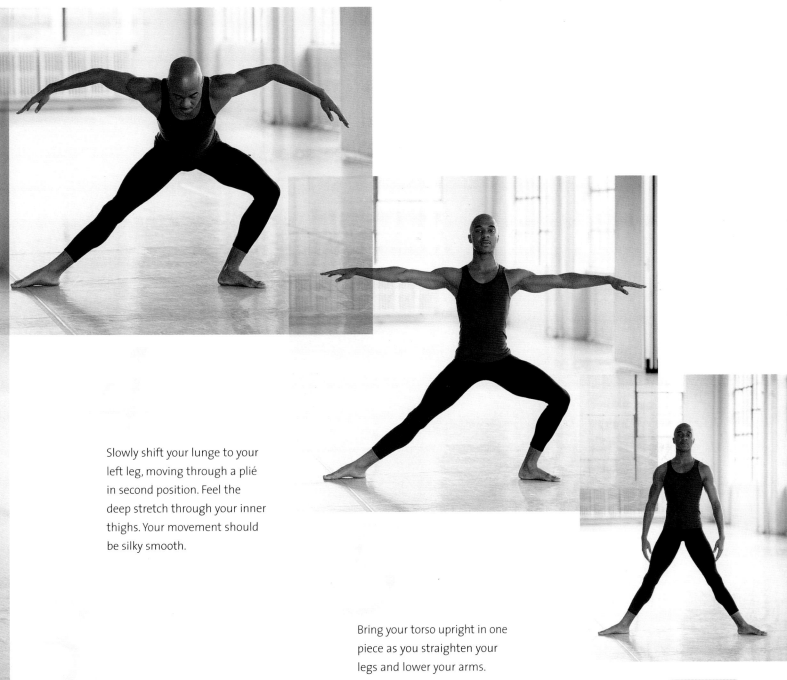

Slowly shift your lunge to your left leg, moving through a plié in second position. Feel the deep stretch through your inner thighs. Your movement should be silky smooth.

Bring your torso upright in one piece as you straighten your legs and lower your arms.

Next tilt your torso forward from your hips so it's at a diagonal. As you tilt your torso, raise your elbows slightly so your arms look like a bird's wings in flight. Your abdominals should be lifted and your neck long.

Repeat the sequence, starting with a lunge into your left leg. This exercise calls for a lot of balance and coordination. Take plenty of time to feel each shape. Once you become comfortable, you can play with the tempo. Repeat four times.

Revelations

Alvin Ailey's *Revelations,* a rousing piece set to a suite of
African-American spirituals, has been seen by more people
than any single modern dance work since its creation in
1960. Ana Marie Forsythe, chairperson of The Ailey School's
Horton department and codirector of The Ailey School-
Fordham University B.F.A. program, reveals the source of
one of this dance's most iconic images.

"Alvin used a lot of Lester Horton's technique in his choreography, and used it dramatically and artistically. He readily
admitted this was how some of his work was inspired. One
day, when we were still in the studios at 1515 Broadway,
Alvin came in and watched me teach for a very long time.
I was teaching Prelude #3, one of the early Horton studies
created in the 1940s. In this study there are those wonderful
Revelations arms. The dancer looks like a bird of prey hovering
low to the ground. When I had finished and the students
had performed it a couple of times, Alvin looked at me and
said, 'That's where I got those arms!' Fortunately, I was on
the ball and replied, 'But you made them famous!'"

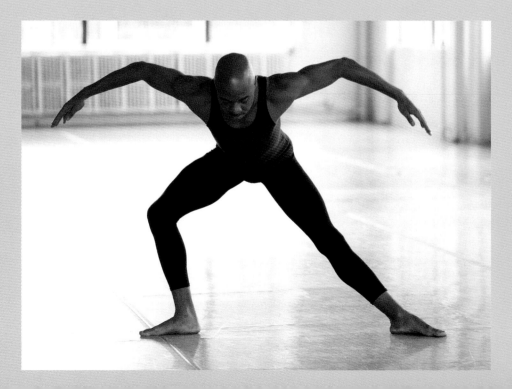

Cool It

If you have ever watched a marathon (or participated in one), you know that when the runners cross the finish line, they don't simply lurch to a dead stop. They slow down gradually, coming to a standstill only when their breathing has returned to normal. This process is known as cooling down. You can think of cooling down as the complement to warming up. Like your warm-up, it is an important transitional activity. A careful warm-up takes you from a sedentary state to one where you are physically and mentally prepared for full-out movement. An effective cool-down in turn facilitates a smooth, safe transition from high activity to relative stillness.

When you're exercising vigorously, your blood rushes to your muscles. Every time your muscles contract, they act like pumps, pushing your blood back up to your heart. A sudden stop can halt this pumping action abruptly; the blood that has been coursing through your muscles may pool in your extremities, which can lead to discomfort or dizziness.

The simplest way to cool down is to lower the intensity and pace of your exercise bit by bit. Gradually make your movements smaller and slower until you sense your heart rate and breathing returning to normal—between two and five minutes. After that you should do some gentle stretches to help relax your still-warm muscles and increase their flexibility.

the dancer's life

Matthew Rushing and Renee Robinson

I like classical music to relax. I love the piano, the Spanish guitar, and rock and roll.
I love fado. I heard it for the first time when we went to Portugal. Being in the Ailey
company has exposed me to so much. *[RR]*

I love music in general—gospel music, classical music, especially Rachmaninoff. I am
crazy about anything with a strong beat: club music, popular R & B. Stevie Wonder is
one of my favorites. *[MR]*

Whatever you're doing—whether taking classes or eating lunch—remember that
you're not doing it just for today. You're doing it for the health of your instrument,
for your future. *[RR]*

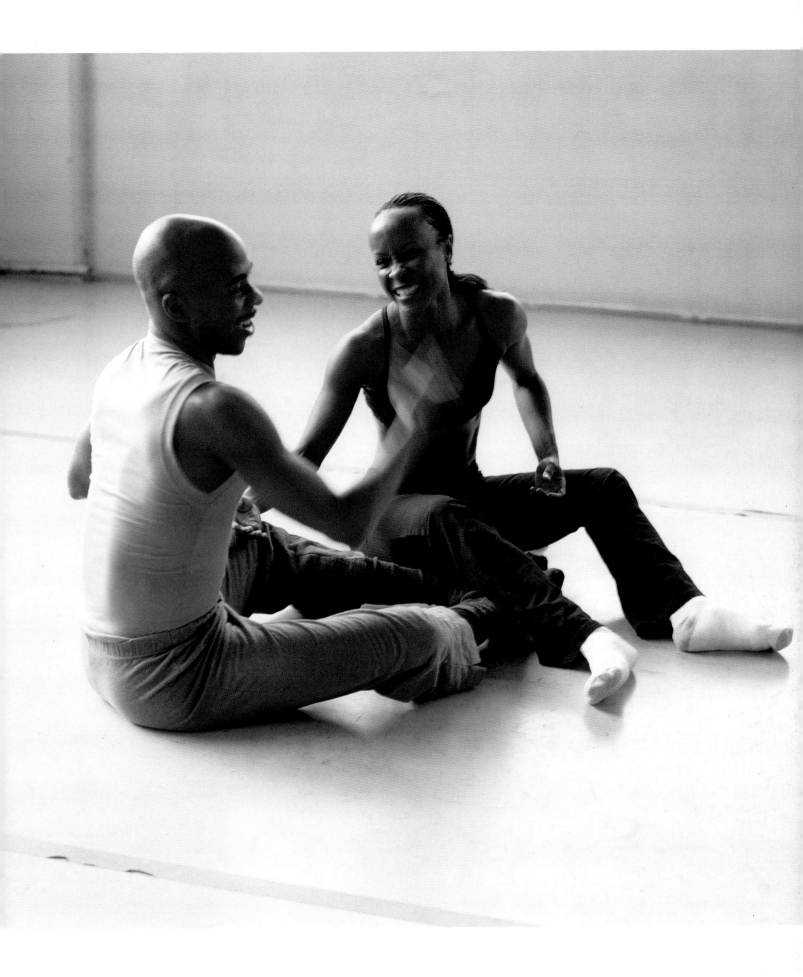

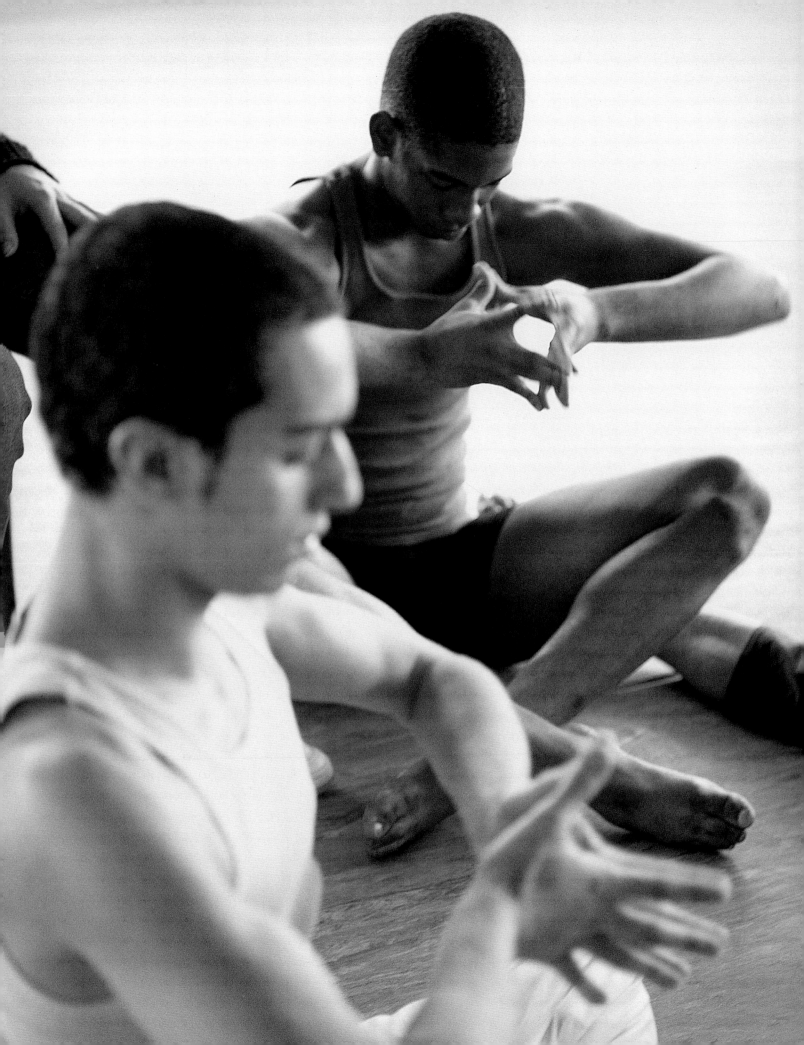

Relaxation and Rejuvenation

While exercising is undeniably stimulating, it is equally important to allow ample time for more relaxing and rejuvenating activities. Your muscles—and psyche—will thank you for it.

There are many tried-and-true methods that help you relax, get control of your breathing, and ease tension throughout your body, face, and mind. The exercises below may be sequenced according to your needs and preferences. You may enjoy pairing a deep breathing exercise with an isolation exercise, for example. Each relaxing exercise is also highly effective when practiced on its own. Try these anytime you need a mental or physical time-out, or want to stave off stress or anxiety.

Relaxation and rejuvenation exercises can be incorporated into your postworkout cool-down, along with some simple stretches (see pp. 87). If you stop abruptly at the end of a vigorous routine without making a gradual transition to stillness, you will feel overheated and, soon, your muscles will become quite stiff.

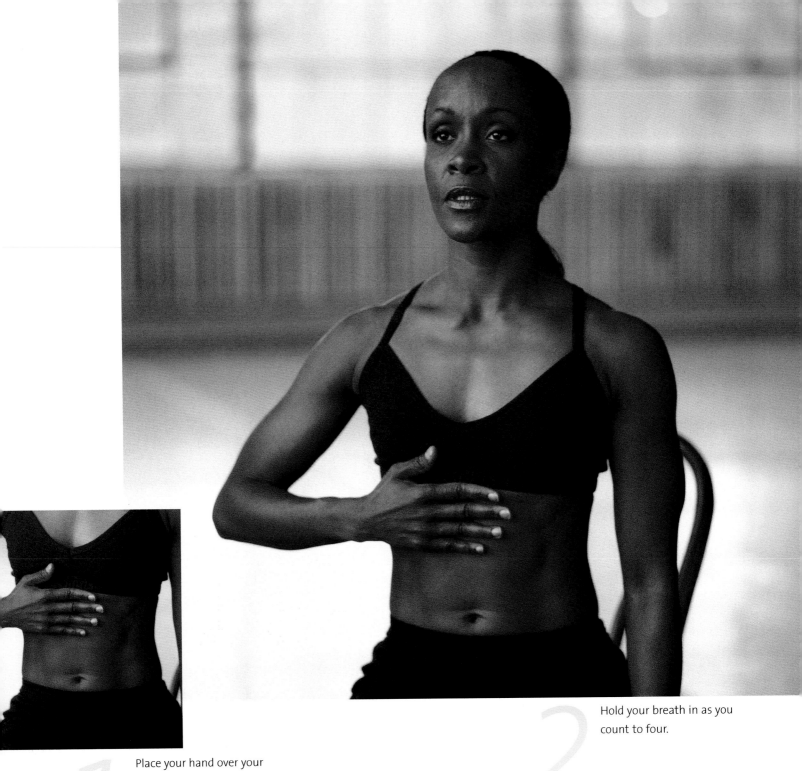

2 Hold your breath in as you count to four.

1 Place your hand over your abdomen and inhale slowly and deeply through your nose. As you inhale, feel your abdomen expand like a bellows as your diaphragm (the large muscle that runs between your chest and abdomen) pushes down on it.

Breathe Easy

When you are feeling anxious or stressed, your breathing tends to become rapid and shallow; your breath is caught high in your chest and throat. As every dancer knows, this breathing pattern quickly exhausts your muscles—they're not receiving ample oxygen—and actually increases your stress.

Diaphragmatic breathing—inhaling deep, restorative breaths through your nose and exhaling through your mouth—prevents hyperventilation, calms a too-rapid heartbeat, and transports healing oxygen to your muscles.

You can practice breathing easily while you're sitting, standing, or lying down.

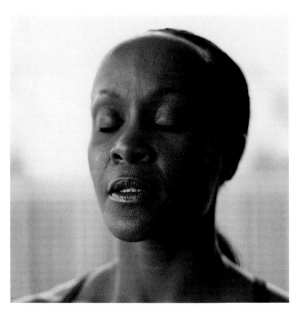

3 Then exhale slowly, through gently pursed lips. Feel your abdomen contract and your face, neck, shoulders, and torso relax.

Repeat several times.

HINT Pay attention to the sound of your breathing and to the calming feelings it generates in your body. Practice this easy breathing regularly, and you'll soon find yourself using it automatically, whenever you need to stave off a sense of panic or decompress from a stressful situation.

Loosen Up

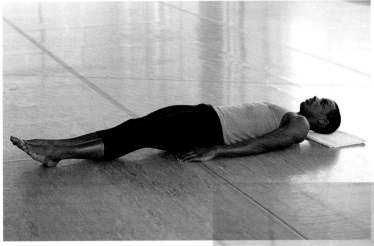

1

Lie down on your back and let your body sink into the floor. Imagine you're a limp, overcooked noodle or a puddle of melting snow. Make any necessary adjustments to your limbs and head for comfort.

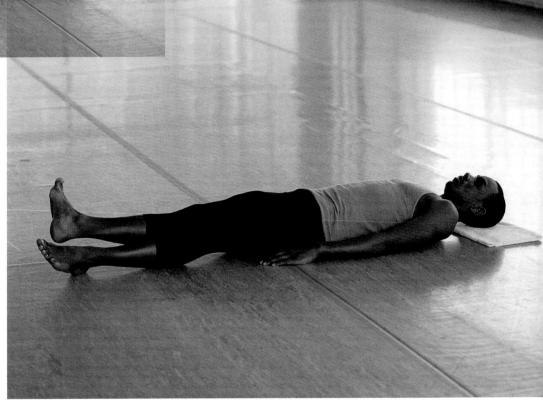

2

Starting with your right leg, flex your toes toward the ceiling and lift your leg a few inches off the floor. Try to keep the rest of your body relaxed.

3

Hold this position until the trembling starts—about 10 to 15 seconds—then tell your leg muscles to release and allow your leg to drop. Feel the tension drain away.

This fail-safe series of exercises involves consciously tensing your muscles, then commanding them to release. This enhances your blood flow and helps clear your mind of anxiety-producing static. You may want to place a small pillow, towel, or rolled-up sweater under your head.

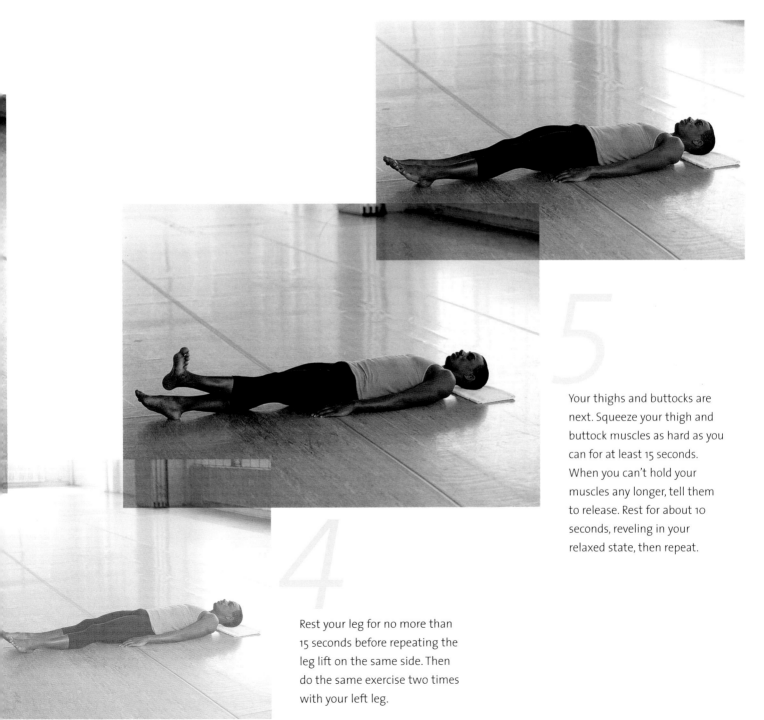

5

Your thighs and buttocks are next. Squeeze your thigh and buttock muscles as hard as you can for at least 15 seconds. When you can't hold your muscles any longer, tell them to release. Rest for about 10 seconds, reveling in your relaxed state, then repeat.

4

Rest your leg for no more than 15 seconds before repeating the leg lift on the same side. Then do the same exercise two times with your left leg.

CONTINUED >

Loosen Up

8

When you are finished, rest a moment before rolling onto one side and slowly getting up.

7

Stretch your arms over your head, clench your fists, and hunch your shoulders up to your ears. Your arms should be raised a few inches off the floor. Hold the contraction for at least 15 seconds, then tell your muscles to release and let your arms drop to the floor. Rest for a moment, feeling the heat flood your muscles, then repeat.

6

Then move on up to your abdominals. Tense your stomach muscles and try to feel the contraction from just below your ribs to just above your pubic bone. Hold for about 15 seconds before telling your stomach to release. Repeat one time.

Facial Tension
You Don't Have To Grin and Bear It

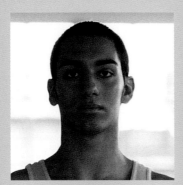
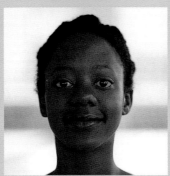
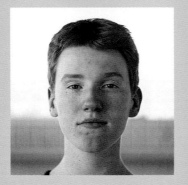

Your face has more than 50 muscles. Your eyelids weigh in with an impressive 12. That's an astonishing number of sites for tension to develop, potentially creating a ripple effect of stress and strain that inevitably migrates to your skull, neck, shoulders, and quite possibly your entire body. Habitual jaw-clenching, for example, can lead to sore molars and tight, throbbing muscles in your neck and at the base of your skull. A constantly furrowed brow could spur debilitating headaches.

Facial tension may be caused by any number of emotions—anger, anxiety, and sadness are among the main culprits. It may also stem from chronic pain, poor posture, eye strain, and dental problems. Although some of these causes require medical intervention, the following exercise focuses on tension that can be alleviated through exercise and relaxation. The first step is to become aware of any facial habits that may be causing you strain or discomfort. Then you can begin to alter those patterns.

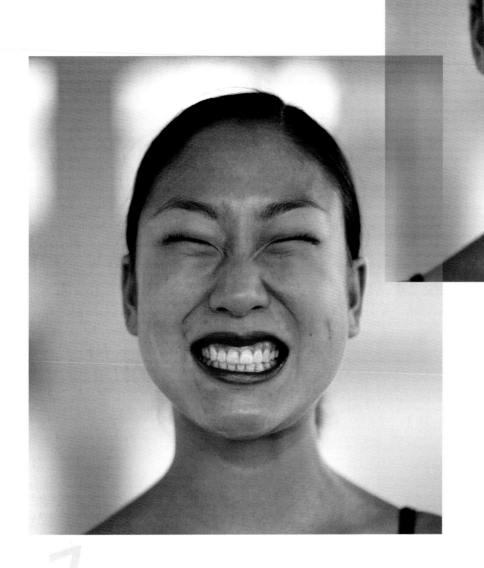

Purse your lips into an extreme cartoon smooch, hold it a moment, then let go. Rest a few seconds, then repeat three to four times.

1

Make a huge jack-o'-lantern grin, hold it for a moment, then release your lips and cheeks until your mouth goes slack. Repeat three to four times.

Face Time

You may perform these exercises while you're sitting, standing, or lying down.

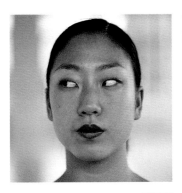

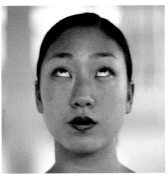

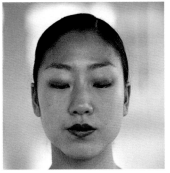

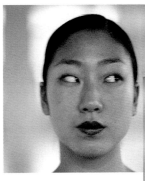

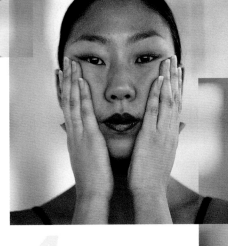

3

Keep your head centered and still as you roll your eyes to your right, up, left, and down. Really look in each direction. Reverse the roll, rest, then repeat three to four times.

4

Massage your jaw, cheeks, and forehead with your hands, then close your eyes and place your palms over your eyes. Relax in that position for a moment.

Get Moving

Sometimes the best way to wind down is to rev up.

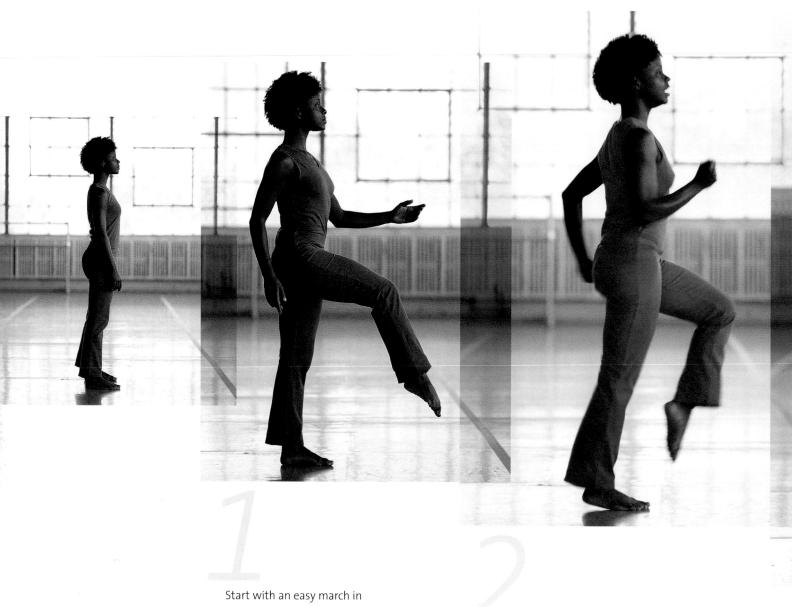

1 Start with an easy march in place at a moderate pace. Let your arms swing in natural opposition to your legs.

2 Begin to raise your knees higher as you step, and start to pump your arms.

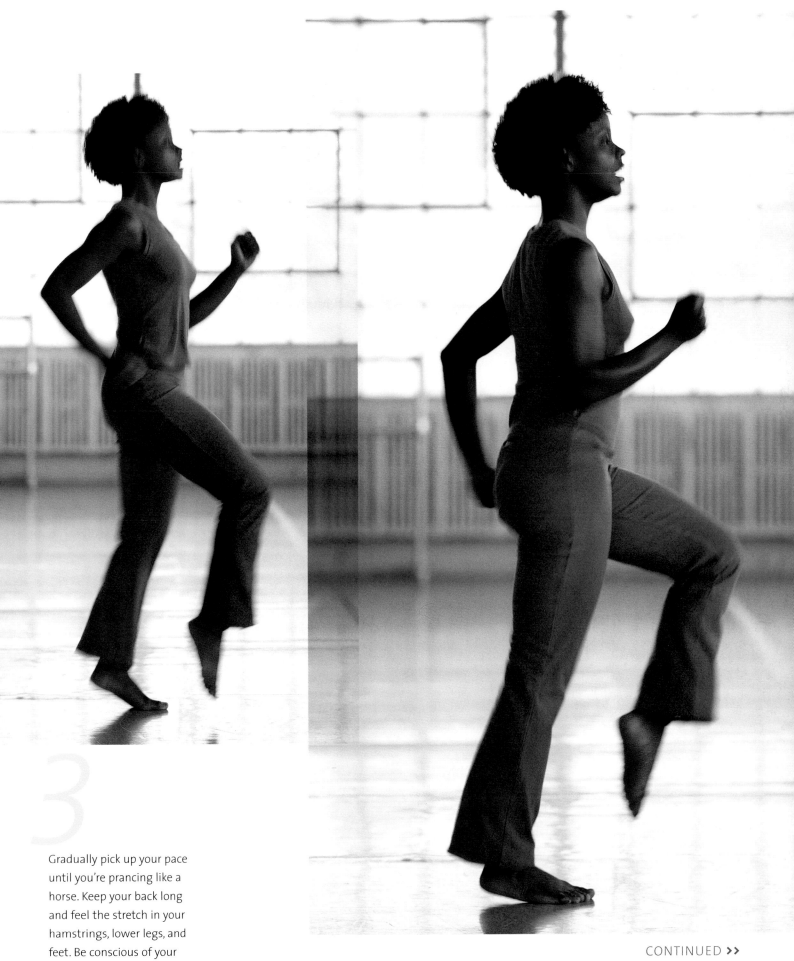

3

Gradually pick up your pace until you're prancing like a horse. Keep your back long and feel the stretch in your hamstrings, lower legs, and feet. Be conscious of your breathing.

CONTINUED >>

Get Moving

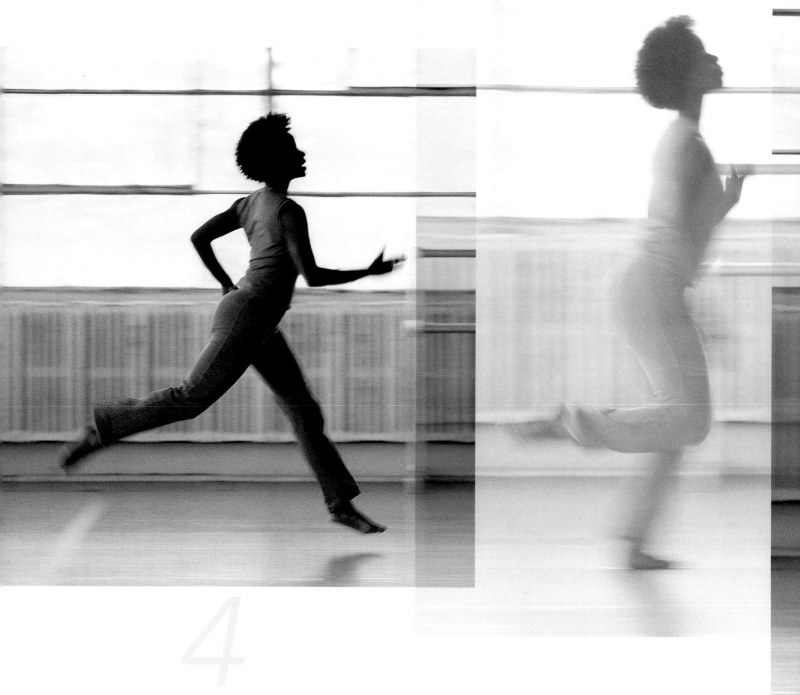

4

If you like, and if you have the
space, turn your prance into an
easy, leaping lope around the
room. Stretch your legs and
allow your arms to swing in
wide arcs.

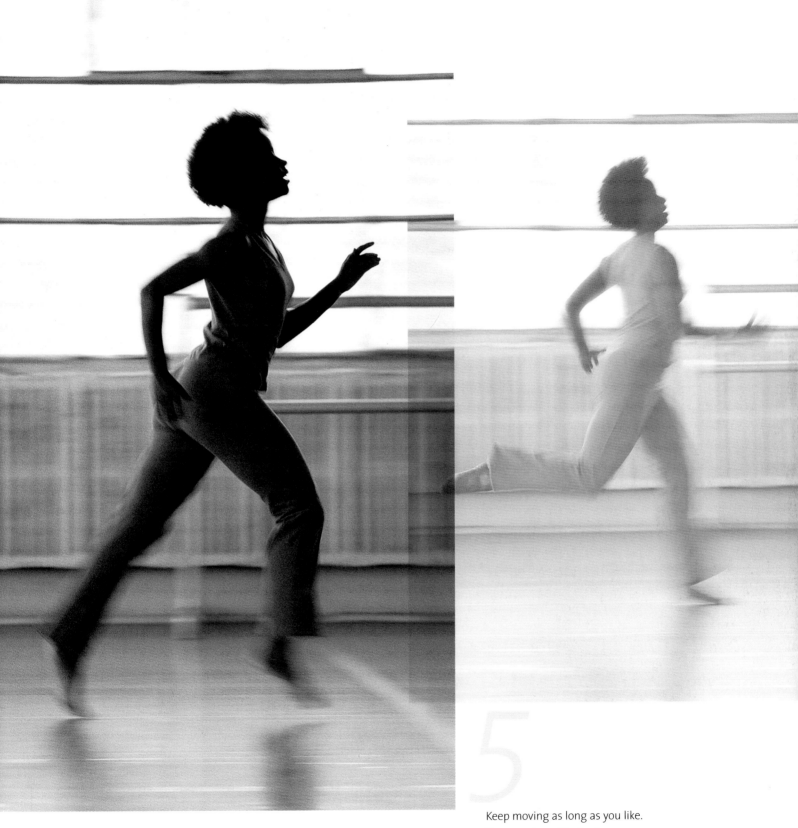

5

Keep moving as long as you like.
You can play with the tempo
and the size of your strides.

CONTINUED >

Get Moving

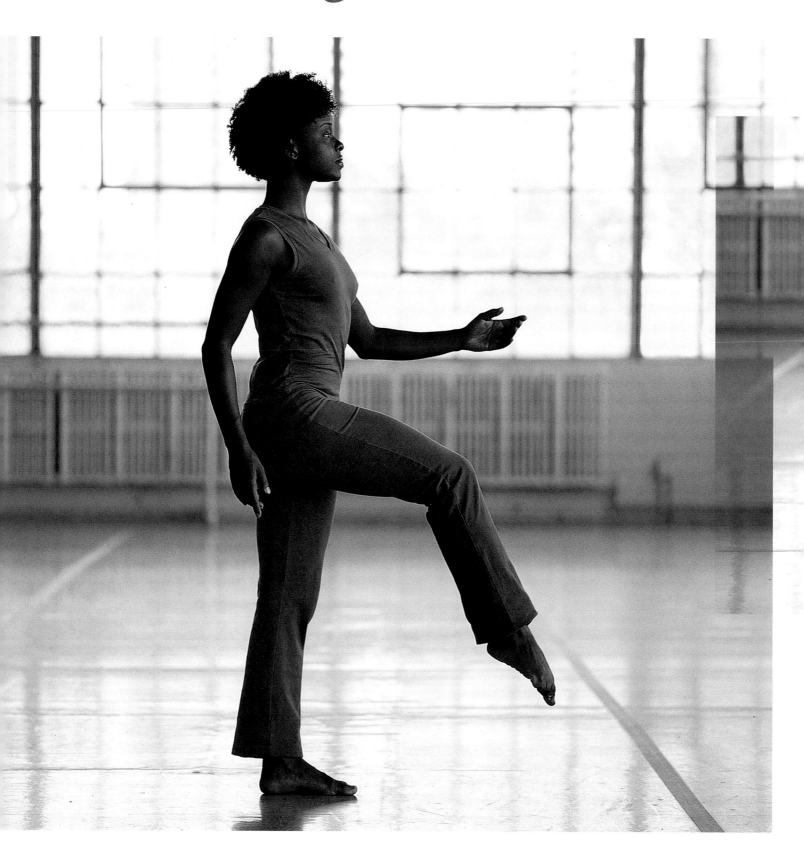

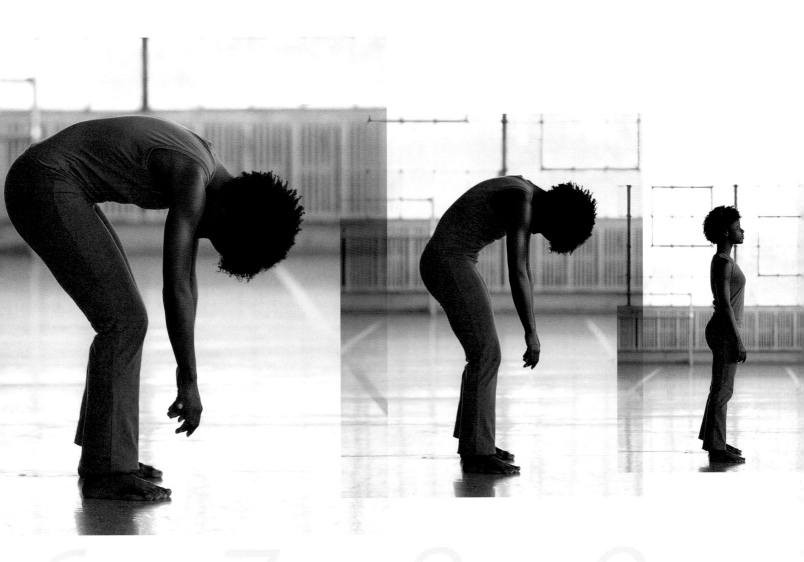

6

When you're ready to stop, slow down until you've returned to an easy march in place. Gradually make your movements smaller and softer until you are standing still.

7

Next, inhale deeply, then exhale as you drop your torso forward until your head hangs over your slightly bent knees.

8

Relax for a moment in this position. Feel the warming stretch in your spine, neck, and along the backs of your legs.

9

Roll up slowly, vertebra by vertebra, starting with your lower back, then torso, upper back, shoulders, and head. You should be in an upright position again.

Tune In to Yourself

Many dancers find meditation extremely calming and physically restorative. There are many effective techniques. The simple method described below is derived from yoga.

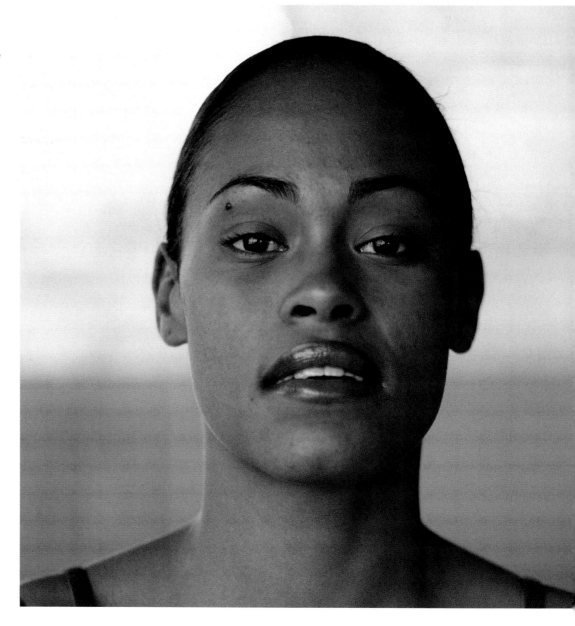

1

Sit up with a long back and neck in a chair or on the floor, whichever is the most fidget-free position for you. Take several deep breaths(see Breathe Easy, page 178) to quiet your body and promote a relaxing frame of mind.

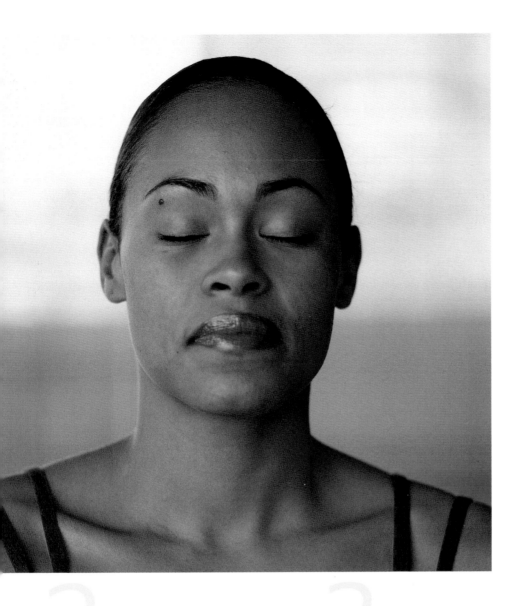

Try to keep your mind tuned in to your breath. If you find your thoughts straying (and they most certainly will), gently steer them back to your breathing. Keep this up for five to ten minutes. As you become more expert at focusing on your breathing, you'll be able to increase your meditation time.

2

When you're ready, close your eyes and inhale again, deeply through your nose, then exhale.

3

Concentrate on your breathing: Cool air moving in, warm air rushing out. If you're having trouble establishing a smooth rhythm, you may wish to count silently as you breathe: Inhale, 2, 3; exhale, 2, 3; inhale, 2, 3; exhale, 2, 3.

You may find that "tuning in" once a day for fifteen minutes; say, early in the morning, can clear the mental cobwebs and help you to focus your thoughts and energy. Or you might prefer shorter sessions, one upon rising and the other just before sleep. Whatever you do, don't get anxious about adhering to a schedule. Even if you manage a session just once a week, you'll still derive benefits. One of the many wonderful virtues of meditation is that there is no one way to practice. Feel free to experiment.

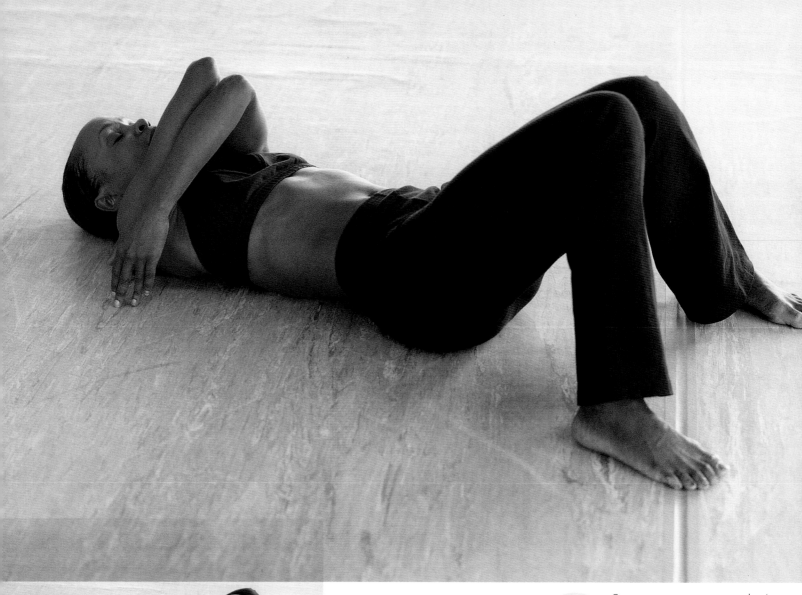

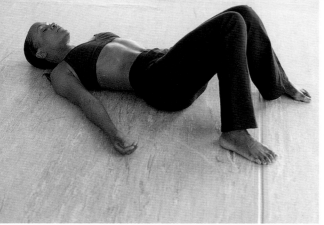

Cross your arms over your chest, allowing your lower arms and hands to hang freely. Again don't pull, push, or hold. Find an easy position. Be conscious of the base of your neck and lower back. Both should be relaxed and resting on the floor. Close your eyes and inhale and exhale deeply, evenly, and slowly.

Lie on your back with your knees bent comfortably at about a 45-degree angle and the soles of your feet flat on the floor. You should open your feet wide enough so that your knees can rest easily against each other. Find a position as free of strain as possible; you don't want to have to hold your legs in place.

Constructive Rest

No, it's not an oxymoron: Rest can be constructive. This dancer's favorite is extremely simple and wonderfully restorative. You may want to place a small pillow, towel, or rolled-up sweater under your head.

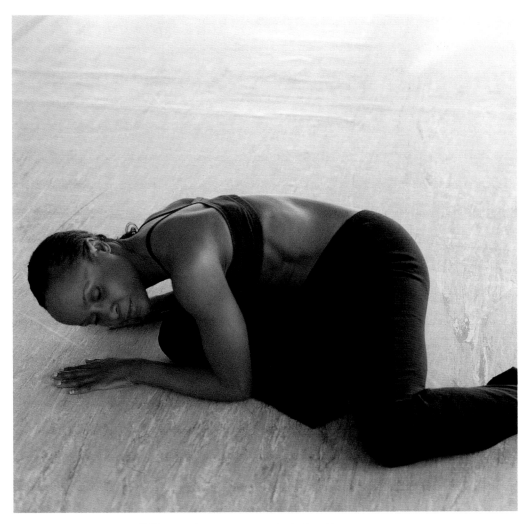

3 When you are ready to face the world, uncross your arms, roll to one side, and get up slowly.

HINT Although it may take a few sessions of constructive rest—it takes work to relax!—soon you will feel your hip and shoulder joints relaxing and releasing.

I like to be prepared: go home and rehearse a movement, listen to the music, learn cues so I know what happens when.

healthy habits
and disciplines

If you are sore, you must evaluate the soreness. Is it because you're trying something new or have you pulled something?

I tend to eat a pretty healthy diet: salads, vegetables, fruit. But every once in a while I break down and have a cheeseburger and fries. I'm only human!

I meditate to let go of tension.

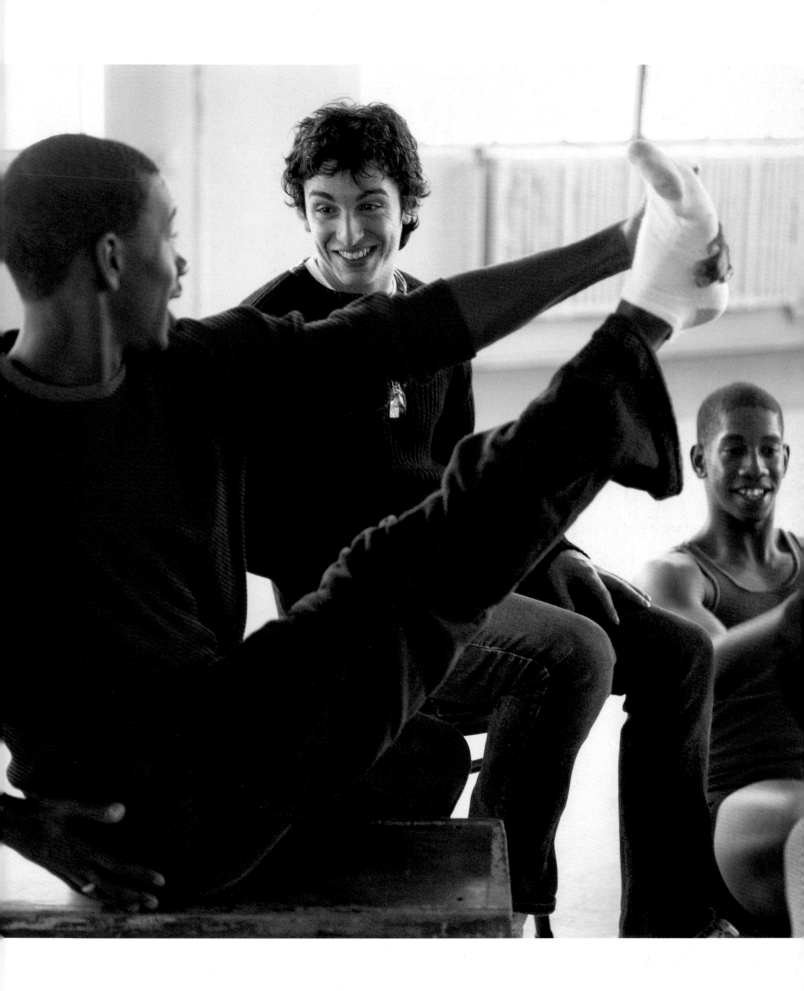

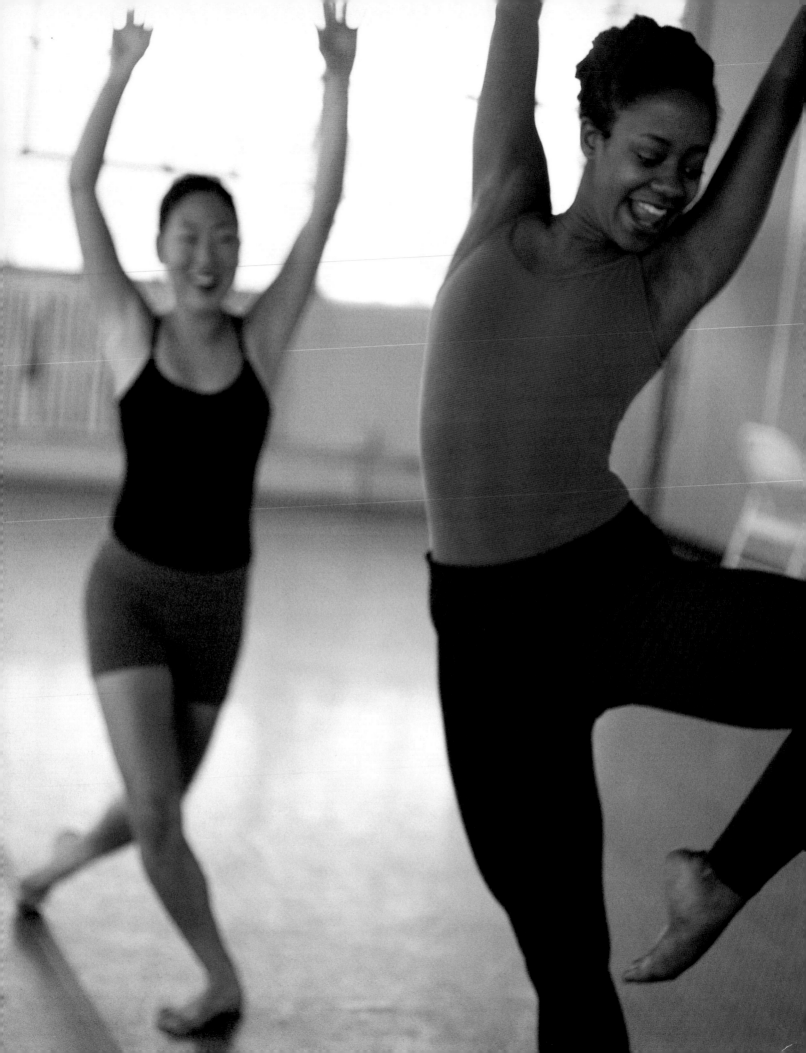

The Music Made Me Do It!

Well, it certainly can help you do it. Whether putting your abs through their paces or executing a space-gobbling movement phrase, the right music can make all the difference. It's no surprise that dancers are particularly sensitive to music. They have strong opinions about what works and what definitely does not. What follows is a list of musical favorites from dancers, Ailey School teachers, and students, as well as selections from Alvin Ailey American Dance Theater's active repertory. This impressive mix of artists and genres will help you make the most of your exercise routine.

DANCERS' FAVORITES

ARTISTS

Ani DiFranco

Billy Holiday

Björk

Bob Marley

Branford Marsalis

Dave Matthews Band

Ella Fitzgerald

Enya

Erykah Badu

Harold Maxwell and the Blue Notes

India.Arie

Jay-Z

Jill Scott

Lauren Hill

Lenny Kravitz

Marvin Gaye

Michael and Janet Jackson

Miles Davis

Mos Def

Musiq Soulchild

Prince

Rachmaninoff

Radiohead

Sarah McLachlan

Stevie Wonder

Talib Kweli

Teddy Pendergrass

Tracy Chapman

Tweet

U2

Usher

Wynton Marsalis

GENRES

"Any and all love songs"

"Piano music of all kinds"

Classical music

Deep house music

Electronic

Gospel

Jazz

R&B

Traditional spirituals and blues

THE AILEY SCHOOL TEACHERS SUGGEST

J.S. Bach, especially The Goldberg Variations

Antonio Vivaldi

Gabriel Fauré

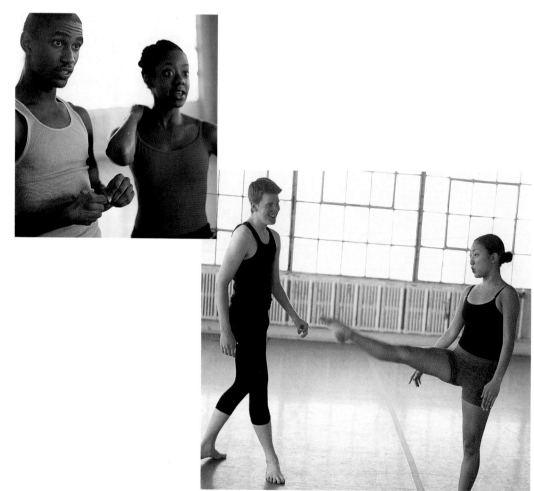

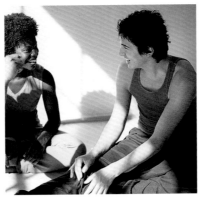

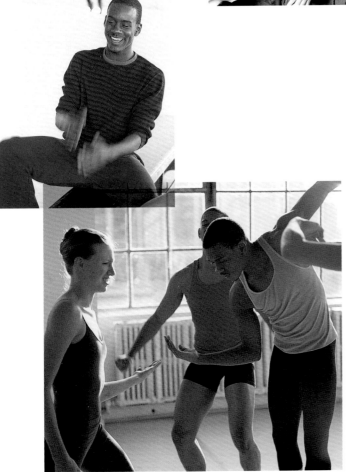

SELECTIONS FROM THE ALVIN AILEY AMERICAN DANCE THEATER REPERTORY

Alice Coltrane, "Something About John Coltrane," *Cry*, choreography by Alvin Ailey, 1971

Antonio Carlos Scott, *Chocolate Sessions*, choreography by Dwight Rhoden, 2000

Branford Marsalis, *Serving Nia*, choreography by Ronald K. Brown, 2001

Charlie Parker, *For "Bird"—With Love*, choreography by Alvin Ailey, 1984

Chuck Griffin, *Cry*, choreography by Alvin Ailey, 1971

Count Basie, *For "Bird"—With Love*, choreography by Alvin Ailey, 1984

Dizzy Gillespie, *For "Bird"—With Love*, choreography by Alvin Ailey, 1984; *The Winter in Lisbon*, choreography by Billy Wilson, 1992; *Serving Nia*, choreography by Ronald K. Brown, 2001

Donny Hathaway, *Sweet Bitter Love*, choreography by Carmen de Lavallade, 2000

Duke Ellington, *The River*, choreography by Alvin Ailey, 1970; "Night Creature," *Ailey Celebrates Ellington*, choreography by Alvin Ailey, 1974; "Black Beauty," "Maha," "The Shepherd," "John Hardy's Wife," "Creole Love Call," *The Mooche*, choreography by Alvin Ailey, 1975; *Grace*, choreography by Ronald K. Brown, 1999

Fela Anikulapo Kuti, *Grace*, choreography by Ronald K. Brown, 1999

Jay "Hootie" McShann and Walter Brown, *Opus McShann*, choreography by Alvin Ailey, 1988

Jerome Kern, *For "Bird"—With Love*, choreography by Alvin Ailey, 1984

Junior "Gabu" Wedderburn, *Shelter*, choreography by Jawole Willa Jo Zollar, 1988

Keith Jarrett, "Runes—Solara March," *Memoria*, choreography by Alvin Ailey, 1979

Laura Nyro, "Been On a Train," *Cry*, choreography by Alvin Ailey, 1971

Laurie Anderson, *Bad Blood,* choreography by Ulysses Dove, 1984

Leon Russell, *A Song for You,* choreography by Alvin Ailey, 1972

Michael Kamen, based on Duke Ellington themes, *Caravan,* choreography
by Louis Falco, 1976

M'Benba Bangoura, *Serving Nia,* choreography by Ronald K. Brown, 2001

Miguel Frasconi, *Following the Subtle Current Upstream,* choreography by
Alonzo King, 2000

Mikel Rouse, *Vespers,* choreography by Ulysses Dove, 1986

Miloslav Kabelac, "Eight Inventions, Opus 45," *Streams,* choreography,
Alvin Ailey, 1970

Mio Morales, *Dance at the Gym,* choreography by Donald Byrd, 1991

Miriam Makeba, *Following the Subtle Current Upstream,* choreography by
Alonzo King, 2000

Patrice Sciortino, "Les Cyclopes," *Hidden Rites,* choreography by Alvin Ailey,
1973

Peter Gabriel, *Bad Blood,* choreography by Ulysses Dove, 1984;"Passion,"
Prayers from the Edge, choreography by Lynne Taylor-Corbett, 2002

Robert Ruggieri, *Double Exposure,* choreography by Judith Jamison, 2000;
Episodes, choreography by Ulysses Dove, 1987

Rolf Ellmer, *Apex,* choreography by Francesca Harper, 2002

Roberta Flack, *Sweet Bitter Love,* choreography by Carmen de Lavallade,
2000

Roy Brooks, *Serving Nia,* choreography by Ronald K. Brown, 2001

Roy Davis, *Grace,* choreography by Ronald K. Brown, 1999

Steve Reich, *Treading,* choreography by Elisa Monte, 1992

Wynton Marsalis, *Here. . . Now.,* choreography by Judith Jamison, 2001

Zakir Hussain, *Following the Subtle Current Upstream,* choreography
by Alonzo King, 2000

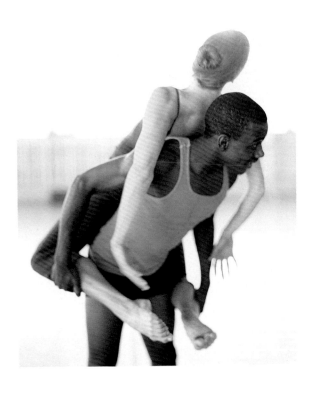

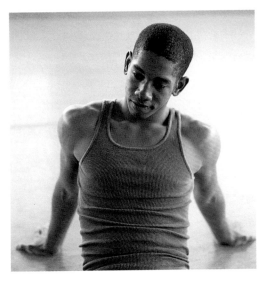

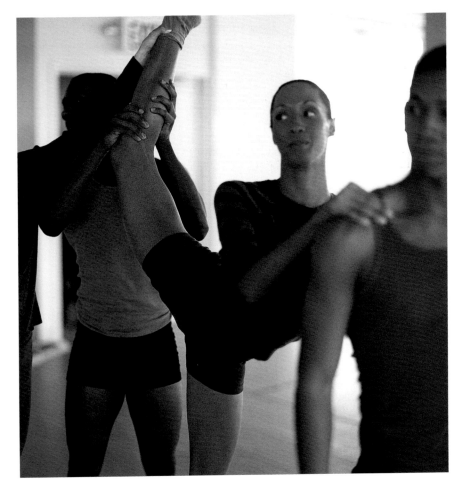

The Ailey School

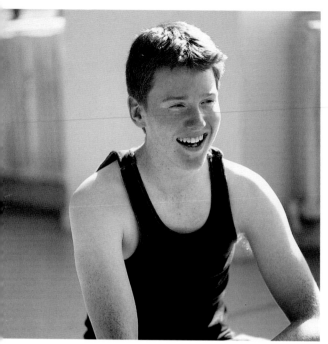

STEVEN McMAHON, CERTIFICATE PROGRAM

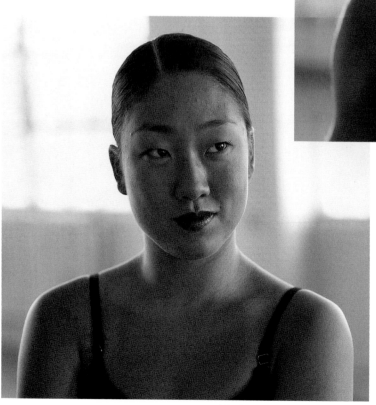

JAMES PIERCE AND COURTNEY CORBIN, B.F.A. PROGRAM

JULIE FIORENZA, B.F.A. PROGRAM

Ailey II
2002-2003 Season

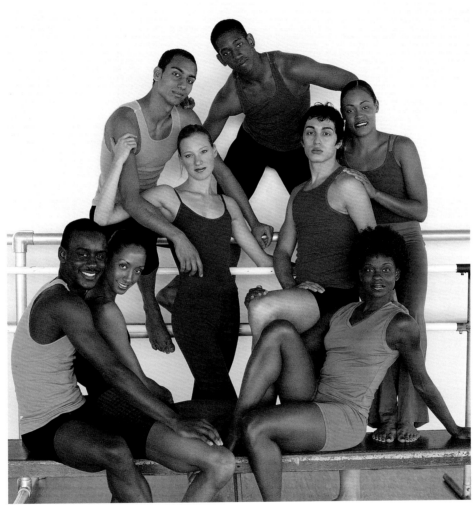

FRONT: KIRVEN J. BOYD, KRISTINA MICHELLE BETHEL, AND BRANDYE LEE.
BACK: ROBERT HALLEY, KATHERINE HORRIGAN, ZACH L. INGRAM, WILLY LAURY, AND HOLLY ALEXIS HYMAN.

Alvin Ailey American Dance Theater

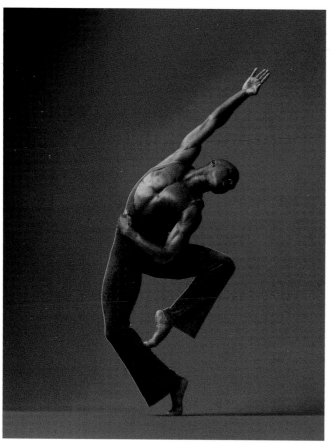

MATTHEW RUSHING IN LOVE SONGS

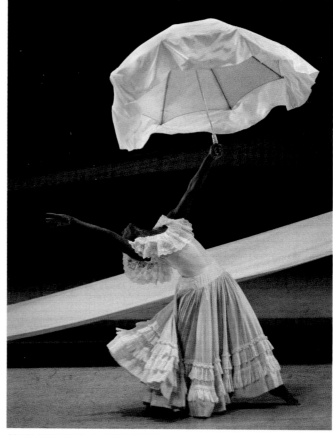

RENEE ROBINSON IN REVELATIONS

All About Ailey

ALVIN AILEY® AMERICAN DANCE THEATER was founded in 1958, and has performed in 71 countries on 6 continents for an estimated 19 million people. The Company has 31 of the most talented and versatile dancers in the world, many of whom are graduates of The Ailey School. A typical season includes tours through the United States and abroad and a New York City engagement at City Center in December.

AILEY II was founded in 1974 to help talented students from The Ailey School make the leap from the studio to the stage. Ailey II has emerged as a professional company in its own right. It has received critical acclaim for its national tours and its residencies at public schools and community centers throughout the United States.

THE AILEY SCHOOL, the official school of AAADT, offers to students of all ages more than 200 classes weekly. The diverse curriculum attracts the most talented dance students from around the world. Founded in 1970, the School offers professional training programs, open classes for adults, and programs for children. The School has partnerships with The Actors Studio/New School and the Professional Performing Arts School in New York, and currently offers a B.F.A. degree in conjunction with New York City's Fordham College at Lincoln Center.

ARTS-IN-EDUCATION & COMMUNITY OUTREACH: In fulfillment of Alvin Ailey's long-standing dictum, "dance is for everybody," the Ailey organization is committed to bringing dance to people worldwide. Its innovative arts-in-education programs include special performances, lecture/demonstrations, technique classes, and curriculum-based residencies. The various activities are designed to develop confidence, discipline and creativity while fostering an appreciation for the joy of dance.

For more information on the Alvin Ailey® Dance Foundation: **www.alvinailey.org.**